The Youngest Bee
A Louisiana Story of Sisterhood, Strength, and Alzheimer's

Virginia Evans

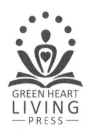

GREEN HEART
LIVING
— PRESS —

ISBN Paperback: 978-1-954493-85-8

Published by Green Heart Living Press

Cover Art by Elizabeth Dyer

Author Photo by Charlotte Purser Arnold

Cover Design by Elizabeth Dyer and Elizabeth B. Hill

Graphics used with permission:

'Bumble Bee Trail' by Leanna Fulanna's Images via Canva.com

'Bees and honeycomb Beehive' by lifeisticac via Canva.com

This is a work of creative nonfiction. The events are portrayed to the best of the author's memory. While all the stories in this book are true, some names and identifying details have been changed to protect the privacy of the people involved.

Dedication

To Caroline Jane and Katherine Margaret,

as namesakes of the Four Bees,

I hope your love and bond as sisters

will always be as close.

The events in this story are told

as I remember them.

As the book explains,

memory is not always reality.

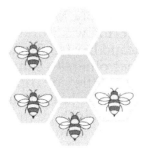

Prologue

IT WAS RIGHT IN the middle of the Market Square, in Colonial Williamsburg, where East and West Gloucester Streets meet, surrounded by tourists admiring the freshly arranged Christmas decorations, when Bill called Peggy a bitch. Well, he actually yelled, "Ever since this trip started, my four sisters have been nothing but bitches to me!" Loudly, in front of a crowd, and of all people—Peggy! Peggy is the sweetest one of all of us. She had probably seldom ever heard the word and surely never said it.

"Bill, I have been nothing but nice to you this entire trip," was the only reply the offended Peggy could muster.

"I said FOUR!" he responded as he stormed off.

We had been in the gift shop looking for a present to give my parents for their 50th wedding anniversary. Since they had been married in November, we had settled on a framed botanical print from the month of November. Peggy had gone outside to ask Bill if he wanted to contribute to the gift and have it be a present from all of us. I'm not sure what else was said, but I'll always remember the day he said all of his sisters were bitches.

It was November of 1992. Instead of a huge golden wedding anniversary party with all their friends, my parents had decided that they wanted a family trip. I had never been on a vacation with my parents and all my siblings before. I had traveled a lot, but never with my whole family. My mother took us on ski trips to Colorado when Katherine was working there, and to Dallas and Ohio to visit Peggy and her family. And every summer, she drove me and sometimes others to summer camp in Virginia. We always took interesting little side trips to parks and shops all along the countryside. But the last actual family trip, one with both of my parents and all their children, was when they all went to Wyoming. Since I was only a fetus in my mother's belly at the time, I don't count that as a family trip for me. So, in November of 1992, at the age of 23, I went on my first family vacation.

I'm not sure exactly why my parents chose Washington D.C. and Williamsburg, Virginia as the destination for their anniversary excursion. But they wanted it, and were mostly glad to have all their children and grandchildren together for a Thanksgiving vacation.

Bill had only been living in Virginia for a few months as he had just recently started teaching computer science at Virginia Commonwealth University. My parents had put him in charge of making the arrangements, despite Katherine having lived there for over a decade. His first mistake was booking a hotel in Washington D.C. that was not on the metro route. This meant having to transport 13 people by car, bus, or taxi to any tourist sites or restaurants. These 13 people ranged in age from three to 73. Not an easy task when you consider the different interests in activities for this age range. The second mistake was booking a tour of the National Archives. I have to admit I was fascinated to see the Declaration of Independence and the Constitution. But after that, I was done and ready to move on. Instead, we were led on a complete tour of the building and into a lecture room where we received what seemed like five hours of information about how our country collects, categorizes, and stores documents. I remember just trying to stay awake, probably fighting off a hangover. Jane's daughters, Elizabeth and Brittany, were only five and three years old. To this day, I don't know how Jane was able to contain them in that room without a single tantrum.

But Bill's worst mistake of the trip had to be the condo situation in Williamsburg, Virginia. After a few days of sightseeing in our nation's capital, the family went on to experience historic

Colonial Williamsburg. Once again, he booked accommodations miles away from all the sights and activities. Because my mother cooked the traditional Thanksgiving dinner (no restaurant could come close to satisfying this family), he booked condominiums rather than hotel rooms. There were three two-bedroom condos for the whole family. These were divided up so the married children each had a condo—one for Peggy, Tim, and their children Aaron and Charlotte, and the other for Jane's family. That left the third condo available for the rest of us, meaning Mom and Dad got a room, Katherine and I shared the room with the twin beds, and Bill slept on the fold-out couch. I'll never forget his first complaint when he learned of this arrangement.

"Every time we go on a family trip, I have to sleep on the couch!" he yelled as he stomped around pouting. Here was this forty-year-old man whining like a small child having to share a toy. I just couldn't help thinking how ridiculous this complaint was since the last family trip had been over 23 years ago!

The condo situation was made worse by the fact that the two condos where Jane and Peggy and their families stayed were in one building at the end of the complex, while the one where Katherine and I stayed with my parents and Bill was in the furthest building from them at the other end. It was probably about a half-mile walk for Katherine and me to go down to visit with our sisters and their families. And, of course, that's where all the fun was.

We all piled up in cars and drove to Colonial Williamsburg. We watched as the costumed employees reenacted the activities of the early colonists. From cobblers to candle makers, it was intriguing to watch the daily activities of people who had lived there over two centuries earlier. We saw the capital and the actual church Thomas Jefferson attended. I have to say that, as a history major, I was fascinated by the feel of the whole place. Along the way, Katherine was making note of the different restaurants and keeping an eye out for a nice place to have dinner on the evening of the actual wedding anniversary.

Back at the condo, my mother began preparations for Thanksgiving dinner. My parents had driven their big conversion van from Baton Rouge, so she was able to bring everything she needed from home to make a huge Thanksgiving feast that was nothing less than what we would have enjoyed at her home.

Katherine and I walked down to Peggy's condo, which had a hot tub. Before long, Jane, Peggy, their husbands, Peggy's children, and I were having a good old time drinking beer in the hot tub. It was great. At some point, even Peggy joined in on the fun, abstaining from the beer, of course. For the first time in the vacation, I think we all really relaxed. At the end of the evening, Katherine and I stumbled back across the long parking lot and into our twin beds in my parents' condo, where Bill was already asleep on the couch.

The next morning, we woke to the smells of Thanksgiving dinner being prepared just as if we were home in Baton Rouge. Imagine my surprise when the first words my parents spoke to me was to scold me for staying out past midnight! Really?! I was 23 years old. I had a college degree. I lived and worked for a company in Dallas, Texas. And was I out barhopping around some strange city? No! I was at another condo in the same complex with my family! Including Katherine, who came home at the same time as me. Was I really getting in trouble for this? Bill was loving it. He couldn't resist chiming in, "Mother, I've been known to have a six-pack of beer in my refrigerator for over a year and never even drink it."

I thought to myself, Loser—*you could use a beer or two with your personality—no wonder no one wants to hang out with you.* But I kept my mouth shut. It was Thanksgiving Day, and the golden wedding anniversary was approaching. I was not going to fight with my parents...or at least, I would try not to make the trip more difficult for them.

That evening, we went back to the hot tub at Peggy's to drink beer. Peggy's husband, Tim, was especially funny and quoting *Dirty Harry* every time he finished a Coors Light. He proudly held up the empty can and stated, "I know what you're thinking. 'Did he fire six shots or only five?' Well to tell you the truth, in all this excitement, I kind of lost track myself. But being that this is a .44 Magnum, the most powerful handgun in the world, and could blow your head clean off, you've got to ask yourself one question: 'Do I feel lucky?' Well do ya, punk?"

Relaxed and drunk, we all just fell out laughing. Then he zoomed the empty "silver bullet" over to the side where we had been stacking empty beer cans into what we eventually called "the beeramid."

That evening, I was careful to make sure that Katherine and I left in time to get home by midnight. Tim offered to drive us and got a good lecture from Peggy about drunk driving, even if it was just to the other end of a parking lot. We walked back and went to sleep in our twin beds.

The Friday after Thanksgiving was the last day of the trip for Peggy and Jane. Katherine and I remained in Williamsburg through Sunday so we could be there for the anniversary dinner on Saturday night. So on Friday, we decided to find a gift for my parents. Wow! Married 50 years. November 28, 1942! We decided on something made locally to commemorate their family vacation and anniversary as well as their marriage. And so we decided on a framed botanical print. Little did we know that choosing this gift and offering Bill the chance to go in on it with us would name our little group and create a closeness among four sisters that would nourish and sustain us through a lifetime.

I don't remember if Bill went in on the gift or not. I don't even know where the print is to this day. But I will never forget that night, back in the hot tub, with more beer, all of us laughing and joking about how all four of us were bitches. And that, of all of us, he said it to Peggy! Of course, she couldn't bear to say the word or even keep hearing it. So, it was shortened to B's. And from then on, we were the four B's. Sometimes, we'd refer to our group as the Four Bees. Since I tend to be blunt, loud, and have no filter, I'm perceived as the meanest, so over time I became the Queen Bee. Our ages may have spanned 22 years, but by being called an ugly word by our brother, we became as close as any four sisters could be.

1

MILDRED LOUISE WALLACE WAS born in 1922 in southwest Louisiana, in a small town in Allen Parish named Kinder. She was the oldest of four children of Ulla and Tillman Wallace. Her father worked for the railroad, and her mother was a teacher. Her absolute favorite activity was reading. By the time she was 15, she had read every book in the school library. They went to church every Sunday, and spent summer evenings on the large wrap-around porch.

After the stock market crashed in 1929, Mildred and her siblings came of age during the Great Depression. But the financial crisis wasn't the worst tragedy of her childhood. When Mildred was only 13 years old, she skipped chores one day to hide in some bushes and read a book instead. From her hiding place she could see her daddy walking home along the sidewalk. A neighbor who had been arguing with her father, and who obviously had some severe mental health problem, walked up to her daddy and shot him. He died right there on the sidewalk while Mildred watched in horror. The neighbor later went home and shot himself. The young, innocent Mildred instantly lost the man she loved most in life and childhood as she knew it was over.

This was a turning event in Mildred's life, without which this story may have turned out differently and the Four Bees might not even exist. Throughout her life, she often referred to the day her daddy was killed. She adored him, and life was not the same for her after he was gone. The event also forever changed the relationship between Mildred and her mother.

Mildred and her brother Charlie were the oldest of Ulla's four children, followed by Bennie (my Uncle Hubert) and Bertie. The way she told the story was, as soon as her daddy's funeral was over, she and Charlie were told to get jobs. Her daddy's income was gone and the family could not live on her mother's teaching salary. They began working anywhere they could and turning their paychecks over to Ulla to spend on the family. Charlie also planted and tended a garden, which supplied the family with fresh fruits and vegetables in the summer and the preserved jarred ones which they saved to eat in winter.

I believe my mother harbored resentment about this situation most of her life. Her stories of her mother were not of the loving generous grandmother I remember. She talked about her mother as a sort of cruel dictator, forcing her to work and taking everything she earned to spend on the younger siblings who did nothing. Now her little brother Charlie was the man of the house, and together, they were forced to grow up fast.

While my older siblings had joyful memories of my grandmother's house in Kinder and I had the loving recollections of time at her apartment when she was much older, my mom seemed to remember no joy from the place. She loved her brothers and sister. And her mother. But as a teenage girl, she could only dream of how to get out and to leave Kinder and her place as a family breadwinner.

Mildred worked hard and studied hard. At the young age of sixteen, she had graduated high school and earned a full scholarship to Louisiana State University. She was elated! Here was her chance. But her mother would have none of it. The family needed Mildred at home to help with money and chores. It took a local councilman to come over and convince Ulla that Mildred was an exceptional student and what a horrible loss it would be for her to turn down this opportunity. He also contacted one of his colleagues at the university and secured Mildred an on-campus job to provide her living expenses. Her mother was finally convinced, and, in the fall of 1938, Mildred was on her way to Baton Rouge, to Louisiana State University and a new future.

2

COMING TO THE CAPITAL city from a small town and being short on funds did not stop Mildred from jumping straight into the college social scene. She came to college with one dress, but she was ready to go. Her first roommate would end up being one of her lifelong best friends, Dorothy "Dot" Colvin (who would later become Dot Howell). In fact, Dot later commented that upon anxiously walking into her dorm for the first time, knowing no one, she immediately knew she would be okay when the first thing she saw was Mildred's Bible on her nightstand. Dot was from Shreveport and not from a poor family like Mildred. She had a full wardrobe, which she readily shared with her roommate, and she was also a member of Phi Mu sorority.

At this time, LSU was considered a military school. The young men participated in ROTC and later entered the military as officers. In fact, LSU produced more officers for World War II than any other institution, including West Point and Annapolis. Referred to as the "Ole War Skule," everyone on campus participated in LSU's support of the military. Mildred served as a "Little Colonel" for the Engineering Regiment. She was also a homecoming maid and a Gumbo Beauty. She had many dates and a full social calendar, but one particular suitor eventually won out.

Mildred was actively campaigning for his opponent in the upcoming election for Class President of the College of Engineering when she first met Red Evans. He was tall and handsome, highly intelligent but with a keen sense of humor, and his most striking feature was his head of thick, red hair. His real name was Williford, but no one ever called him that, except for his mother. Throughout his life, he was known as W.J. "Red" Evans. He was smitten and determined to win her over. Not just to his side of the election, but to win her heart.

Mildred had plenty of dates, but the ones she enjoyed the most were the ones with Red. Once when she was back in Kinder for the Christmas holidays, she wrote to her roommate about the radio she received from him along with her other gifts.

"I just couldn't wait to tell you the good news," she wrote, "We have a radio now & it is really the stuff—ivory & stuff—W.J. sent it to me. This has indeed been a Merry Christmas—Bruce sent me a dozen white carnations, Ed sent me some lovely blue stationery, Mike gave me perfume, and I got just worlds of things. But I think a radio and carnations (I made a beautiful corsage & wore it to a party in Lake Charles last night)—I am just so excited. Write to me. Love, Mildred," followed by "Isn't W. J. wonderful!"

The two were eventually courting and became one of the most popular couples among the LSU graduating class of 1942.

After graduation, most of the boys from the class were enlisted in the armed services and sent to fight overseas. Since the attack on Pearl Harbor on December 7, 1941, some had even enlisted to serve prior to graduation. Red's roommate, Alex Box, a football and baseball star, even took extra classes to graduate early to serve. He was eventually killed at Kasserine Pass, Tunisia, after having been awarded the Distinguished Service Cross in the earlier North African landings for single-handedly knocking out six machine guns and a field gun with grenades. LSU later named its baseball stadium in honor of Alex Box.

Mildred and Red were married on November 28, 1942. They lived together on army bases while he trained in the United States, and a little over a year later, when it was time for him to ship out, they promised to write to each other every day. This promise was kept, and their letters provide keen insight into their relationship with each other as well as their experiences at war in Europe and on the home front. They carefully numbered each letter to each other. They kept up with which chapter of the Bible each was reading, hoping that, just maybe, they were reading the same passage at the same time even though they were half a world apart.

Red served as captain of the Army's 529th Engineer Light Ponton Company, which began its mission at Camp Swift, Texas in February 1943 and eventually built bridges across France, Belgium, and Germany. It was these bridges that allowed Allied troops, artillery, and supplies to make it across Europe and eventually defeat Nazi Germany and bring the war in Europe to an end. As captain, Red led over 200 men in his company, earning their respect along the way. This group of men always remained close and had several reunions for over fifty years after the war was over.

During their time apart, Mildred's and Red's letters often described their plans for the future. They expressed some doubt over their decision to wait until after the war to have children, but agreed they had done the right thing. But they definitely wanted a family. They referred to the future home they would build together in which to raise their four children. That's right, the plan was to have FOUR. They often referred to these future offspring in their letters as "so-high," "junior," and "the twins." And so that was the plan. What's the phrase (or is it a country song?), "You make plans, and you hear God laughing!"

After VE day, the Army had the task of getting all of the soldiers home or to the Pacific. Of course, this would take time and planning. Once the war with Japan ended in August, 1945, it was time to move all the troops back to the United States and home. The way I always heard the story was, each of the men in my dad's company was allowed to send one free telegram consisting of six words or less, letting a loved one know when they would be arriving home. Mildred knew instantly when her husband would arrive when her telegram read, "Buy two tickets to Tulane Game!" And so began Red's LSU home football game attendance streak.

3

ONCE THINGS SETTLED DOWN after the war, Mildred and Red began their plans to raise a family together. Their first child, Margaret Alice (known as "Peggy"), was born in 1947. I guess Peggy was the "so-high" referred to in their war letters. Peggy was followed by William Box (known as "Bill") in 1949. He wasn't named after my dad, but rather his roommate and friend, Alex Box, but I suppose he was the "junior" referred to in the letters. Peggy and Bill were not followed up by twins; however, my parents went on to have my brother Jack Alexander in 1953 and Katherine Louise in 1955. By this time, they were settled in the home they built in Baton Rouge with their four children, and life was just as it should be.

Mildred and Red both went on to earn master's degrees from LSU after the war. Red worked as an architect for a firm, but eventually went on to open his own private practice. Unable to be satisfied with the work of any other secretaries, Mildred became the secretary of his private practice. Although, with her job description and duties, today she would probably be called office manager, CEO, or just the Boss!

But Mildred was not just busy raising children and running an architecture office. She was involved in many clubs and participated in as many social events as possible. She became an outstanding cook and gracious hostess. Their home was the setting for many parties, and their friends seemed to multiply as they had groups from work, church, clubs, LSU, and parent associations. How she managed to fit all her activities into her schedule and still have time for her children is fascinating to me. Yet she made time to sew Halloween costumes and party dresses, drive everyone to their practices and activities, and spend quality time with all her family.

Mildred was also known for the way she celebrated holidays. She went all out when it came to decorations, and these got larger with the years. Christmas not only included a tree, but garlands, figurines, nativity scenes, and later, a complete snow village of ceramic houses that lit up under one of her trees (by this time there were two!) At Easter, she had stuffed bunnies, porcelain bunnies, chicks, and eggs, as well as a small tree of delicate ornaments made from real eggshells covered in soft velvet with an opening showing miniature scenes of tiny figurines inside. Every holiday was a reason to decorate, celebrate, and entertain.

Everything was perfect, and going along just as planned. Until one glitch happened...well, two. But they were good glitches. Six years after Katherine was born, on the day after their 19th wedding anniversary in 1961, Mildred and Red had an unexpected surprise known as my sister, Jane Ellen Evans. Then, just two months before Peggy was to graduate college in May, 1969, I came along! My dad thought he would be funny and call his mama and tell her, "I've really messed up now. I've gone and gotten my secretary pregnant!"

"Oh no! You didn't!" she exclaimed, before remembering that my mom was his secretary.

By then, both of my grandmothers were a little put out that none of their granddaughters had been named after them and wanted me to take their names. Therefore, they argued I was to be either Ulla Ethel or Ethel Ulla. Thank goodness my parents decided to name their sixth child after my dad's grandmother, so I became Virginia Caroline.

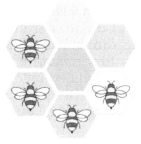

4

Now Mildred and Red had six children over a span of 22 years. Obviously, the house was too small. They had planned on building a new one in a more modern subdivision; however, the lot next door became available, and the decision was made to add on to the existing house. I've been told that while showing my siblings the blueprints for the new addition and describing where each room was to be, they pointed to one room on the plan and announced, "this will be the baby's room."

"What!? Baby!? You can't have ANOTHER baby!" Katherine exclaimed before she stormed off. I guess for her it was bad enough when Jane came along and took her place as the youngest. Now there was going to be another one to add to the mix and chaos of the Evans family.

The addition was thoughtfully designed by Red. Careful to comply with the building restrictions of the subdivision, he designed it to have only a hallway, a stairway landing, and closets taking up the space between the old house and the new part. These areas measured the exact length required between two houses in the neighborhood. That way, someday the two houses could be separated if necessary, without losing any plumbing or living space.

The downstairs consisted of an enormous kitchen (especially for 1969) overlooking a vast family room with a fireplace at the other end. The family room had soaring twenty-foot ceilings and a wall of plate glass windows framing the park-like backyard. There were three pantries and a laundry room fit for a platoon. The upstairs consisted of the master bedroom, my bedroom, and my dad's drawing room. His drawing room remained unfinished most of my life, meaning he worked in a room with plywood flooring surrounded by exposed studs and pink fiberglass insulation. I thought his drawing room was great, and especially loved how he measured all our heights against one of the bare studs as we grew; he carefully wrote our names, heights, and the dates on the bare wood.

The upstairs rooms also had large plate glass windows looking out onto the lawn. My room had a view of the enormous backyard. Each window was framed by gauzy white lace curtains which were rarely closed, but too thin to block any light from the afternoon sun even if they had been. My parents' bedroom and my dad's drawing room had no curtains. At night, our activities must have been seen like watching a fishbowl by all the neighbors and anyone happening by. Friends young and old always commented about how my dad could be seen working at his drawing table until the late hours of the evening through the upper left window of the new house.

The upstairs rooms only covered half of the square feet of the downstairs. My room, the master bedroom, and my dad's drawing room all opened onto a long solid balcony which overlooked the family room. This was one of my favorite features of the house. I could look down at the solid terrazzo floor below and see the long white vinyl couches, the enormous fireplace, and the kitchen counter. If I looked straight ahead from the balcony, I could see the two jumbo white globes hanging from their stems which lit up the family room at night. During the day, I could look out and see the vast green backyard, which ended in groves of fig trees, camellias, and tall water oaks. If I needed to bring dirty clothes to be washed, I could simply toss them over the balcony onto the floor below, then walk downstairs, gather them up, and carry them the short distance to the laundry room.

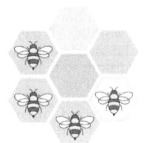

5

ONCE THE ADDITION WAS complete, Mildred had a home ready for some real entertaining. She started buying a Christmas tree which was between 18 and 20 feet tall each year for the family room, as well as a smaller one for the formal living room. Putting up the giant tree required a team effort, meaning all of the family and sometimes neighbors were required to participate in carrying it through the sliding glass door and then lifting it up. Some of us would be on the balcony, pulling on ropes tied to the top of the tree, while others would be downstairs, pushing the bottom of the tree to its proper position on the terrazzo floor below.

Mildred became known for her massive tree and Christmas decorations and was even featured in the "People" section of the local newspaper about it. She hosted Christmas parties for her various clubs, and of course her Sunday School class. The house became the venue for all the reunions for the LSU class of 1942 and several other functions for the university. I'm not even sure how many weddings, receptions, bridal showers, and engagement parties she held there. But the holidays were the most important.

Every time Mildred hosted a party, Jane and I learned the hard way to stay out of her way. The entire day leading up to the party time was stressful. At first, she would be shouting at us to clean this and vacuum that. Then eventually she just wanted us out of the way, along with our toys and any other evidence of our existence. After working all day making the yard look immaculate, Dad would move the television set, rabbit ears and all, up to the master bedroom so that Jane and I could watch it during the party and stay upstairs.

As soon as the first guest arrived, my mother's seemingly bad mood instantly disappeared and she became a gracious and welcoming hostess. Soon, the aroma of the food would drift upstairs and Jane and I would be starving for a plate, which would eventually be brought up to us to eat on the floor of the bedroom in front of the television. Our attention would drift between watching *The Love Boat* and *Fantasy Island* to peering over the balcony to watch the adults at the party. The conversations were too hard to comprehend as we just heard a roar of voices talking and laughing over each other. Eventually, guests would begin to say their goodbyes and thank-yous as they left full and satisfied. Once everyone was gone, my parents would begin cleaning up after the company—only during this type of cleaning, my mom was always in a good mood, laughing as she recalled different stories she had heard during the party.

My favorite of her Christmas parties had to be the one she held annually for her Sunday School class. On the day of the party, members of the class would be in and out all day, dropping off their card tables with their names written on the bottom for identification. Once set up, my mom decorated each table with a red or green square tablecloth and a centerpiece consisting of a lovely porcelain angel surrounded by holly or camellias. I don't know why, but these angels were precious to me and once she unpacked them and placed them on the tables it felt like Christmas was really here. The guests would later return, each carrying a dish which would be set out on the dining room table. Using my mother's Lenox Christmas china, the guests would fill their plates from the buffet style dining table and take a seat at one of the decorated card tables to enjoy their meal. I always loved peeking over the balcony to watch all the guests enjoying each other's company as well as the food and decorations. These parties are the ones which come to my mind when I think of home and Christmas.

It wasn't just the decorations and big parties that made our home special. There was now room enough for everyone to come home for the holidays—not only my older siblings, but aunts, cousins, and grandparents would travel to stay with us. The old part of the house had four bedrooms and a large room across the back which was always called "the old living room." The kitchen was often full of family and friends and smelled of Mildred's excellent cooking. During most days, people would be gathered around the kitchen table talking and laughing. If the chairs were all occupied, there would usually be someone or more, sitting on the kitchen steps taking part in the conversation. And if the group included my Uncle Charlie, Aunt Bertie, or Jack, my mother brought out the ashtrays and cigarette smoke hovered overhead.

And so this is how I grew up. This is how I remember it. Too young to have lived under the same roof with Peggy or Bill as a child. Too young to remember sharing a room with anyone. But always surrounded by people and love.

6

I HAD A DIFFERENT kind of relationship with my parents than my siblings did. For one, they were the same age as most of my friends' grandparents. I was usually proud of this age difference. I remember a teacher in elementary school asking anyone whose grandfather had fought in World War II to raise their hand. I raised my hand proudly, and, when called upon, exclaimed, "my dad fought in World War II!"

"No, that was your grandfather," she replied, insisting that I was mistaken.

"No, I never even met my grandfather. But my dad DID fight in World War II!"

I argued with her and she refused to believe me. The next day I brought pictures of my dad in uniform and some memorabilia of his from the war in Europe to show her. She surely was surprised to find out that I was correct after all.

The only sibling I remember playing with as a child was Jane, and she graduated from high school when I was in fourth grade. I thought everything Jane did was perfect, and I wanted to be just like her. I found a diary I kept in fourth grade and the entries were filled with thoughts like, "Jane had a date with Danny tonight" and "Jane got a new dress." One entry stated that "Jane is at the beach for senior trip" followed by a week of blank entries until she could get home and I could report more about her. I would follow Jane and her friends around and sit outside her bedroom door and try to listen to them. I was such a pest and I can't imagine being in high school and having to put up with this obnoxious little sister. But she's the only sibling I remember growing up in the house with.

Jane did play with me, however. We would ride bikes for hours around the neighborhood, making sure to speed up when we had to pass the spooky-looking house in which the two mean boys who terrorized all the kids in the neighborhood lived. We would go to the neighborhood park together and play on the playground. Sometimes, when the weather was just right, my parents would let us walk home together after Sunday school and skip "big" church.

Later, when Jane could drive, she would graciously take my friends and me to movies, the mall, or sometimes even the water slide (not a water park like they have today—it just had a big slide). I say graciously; however, I'm sure she was threatened by my mother with something much more awful had she refused to drive us around. But she did it, and I am grateful to this day.

I had a best friend in kindergarten who continues to be one of my very best friends. I'm sure she was my dad's favorite out of all my friends because she had red hair! One night, when she was sleeping over and Jane was spending the night out with her friends, we decided to sleep in Jane's bed. The next morning, we discovered that my friend had wet the bed in the middle of the night. I knew this meant serious consequences for her, so my friend and I carefully made the bed (without changing the sheets) and arranged Jane's things as they were, hoping she wouldn't notice. When she got home, she just about screamed when the stench of stale urine hit her as she walked into her room.

"Please, please, please don't tell," I begged her. Jane sympathetically stripped the bed, washed the sheets, and re-made it without telling anyone. We still joke about this today and agree that we owe her big time for putting up with us.

I was likewise the only one of my friends to be an aunt in kindergarten! Yes, at the age of five, I became an aunt when Peggy and Tim had Aaron. It was also strange to have classmates whose parents went to school with my sister, Peggy. I remember that when the World's Fair came to New Orleans in the early 1980s, my parents took Aaron, Charlotte (Peggy and Tim had a daughter two years after Aaron was born), and me to see it. When we got to the ticket counter, I was the only one out of the five of us to need a full price ticket. Both of my parents qualified for the senior discount and my nephew and niece qualified for the under 12 discount. Thus, the age difference in my family made me unique.

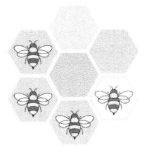

7

As THE YOUNGEST, I believe I spent more time with my parents than most of my siblings. I attended a private elementary school located in downtown Baton Rouge, only a few blocks from my dad's office. My dad often drove me to school on his way to work. After school, my mom would usually be waiting for me outside, and I would walk with her back to the office. There, I would do homework or explore the building until it was time to go home.

My dad's office was on the fourth floor, and we always rode the elevator up. I would push the buttons saying, "Close door, push four," thinking I had invented a clever rhyme to help us always remember where his office was. The stairs were marble, and I would take the coins my mom handed me from her purse and skip down to the second floor to get a Coke and a snack out of the machines. The Coke machine had a long, skinny, door which revealed the tops of the different flavors of Coke (that's what we called all the drinks—Coke—never soda or pop). Once you put in the correct change, you could open the door and pull out the bottle you selected. There were boxes on the side of the machine in which to put your empty bottles when you were done.

There was also a mail slot with a glass front encased in decorative brass which ran from the top to the bottom of the building.

Each floor had a slot through which the sender could drop their outgoing mail and let it fall into the large box on the first floor to be collected by the postman (they always said postman, not mailman). If my mom had outgoing mail to send before leaving for the day, I would make her hold onto it while I ran two floors below so I could watch it fall through the glass on its way down. It's amazing what a thrill I got from the little things when I was young.

As an architect, my father had an exciting office—at least, I thought it was. There were no computers then, so all his work was drawn by hand. His office had a room full of drawing tables and seemingly endless supplies of colored pencils, markers, tracing paper, glue, and any supply you could need to create art projects as a child.

All of the office supplies were purchased from Latil's, the local office supply and stationery store across the street from the office. At the beginning of each school year, they would take the supply list sent home by my teacher and deliver all the items on the list to the office. On occasion, my mom would allow me to walk over there by myself and I was delighted as I spent hours gazing at the things in that shop. Most of the office furniture and big supplies were kept upstairs. Downstairs was more like a Hallmark store. I would gaze for hours at miniature figurines, stickers, cards, gifts, and at Christmastime, Hallmark ornaments. The owners were so nice to let me just gaze for as long as I wanted up and down every aisle. Every now and then I was allowed to pick out a small thing to buy and charge it to my dad's account. They even let me sign my name for it.

The time spent at my dad's office was a treasure and I was fortunate to have that experience and that special time with him. I remember the smell of his pipe smoke combined with Wrigley's gum, pencil shavings and the ditto machine. I still have his briefcase, and sometimes, as a treat to myself, I will open it and just inhale the scent for a few seconds. This can bring back a flood of memories of my parents and my time with them as a child.

8

TO CALL MY DAD a workaholic would be an understatement. He was always at work all day long. His dress shirts had holes in the elbows where he had worn through the fabric from hours of drawing at one of his tables. Recently, I met a younger architect who told me that his first job out of school was working for my dad.

"I'll never forget working there in that drawing room with the other young draftsmen. One Christmas Eve, your father came into the room around 4:30 p.m. and announced to all of us that, since it was Christmas Eve, he decided that we could go ahead and leave before 5!"

I laughed at the story, thinking that if I worked there it would have been hard not to come back with, "Thanks a lot, Ebenezer!"

It seemed like he was never sick and never took a vacation. He would bring work home with him, which he would do in his drawing room after dinner. I vividly remember him coming and going in his suit with his briefcase in one hand and sets of plans or blueprints under his arm. Kissing my mother would be the last thing he did in the morning before leaving for the office and the first thing he did when he got home in the evening. Their college love affair never seemed to fade.

When saying goodbye to me, he always followed up with, "I'll see you in the funny paper!" And when greeting me when he got home it was, "Well, I'm glad you got to see me today!"

I believe my dad's work ethic (or obsession) was something that got into his system from having been through the Great Depression and World War II. I think it caused him to appreciate having work to do and getting paid for doing something he loved. It also created a determination that his family would never have to go without like he did, so he was going to work as hard as possible to provide for them. Not only did these beliefs cause him to work long hours, but they also taught him to conserve and recycle way before anyone was talking about saving the environment. He bought Wrigley's Doublemint or Juicy Fruit gum, but only chewed one half of a stick at a time, carefully putting the second half back in the package to save for later. Supplies, tools, and hardware at the office and at home could be found stored in old baby food jars. After he ate the bagged lunch my mom had made for him, he would carefully refold the bag to bring home so it could be used for lunch the next day.

I believe the Great Depression and World War II had a completely different effect on my mom. Mildred was definitely a shopper! Neither she, nor any of her four girls, were going to go without the nicest clothes she could find. She was known to all the sales ladies in the Baton Rouge small dress boutiques, as well as in the children's boutiques. One of my earliest memories is of her taking me to buy clothes at a small upscale store called T'Nincy. The ladies in there loved when she would come in, probably because they knew she was going to spend. I remember one of them trying to help me to try on the pile of new things my mother had picked out and sent to the dressing room. Refusing any help, I exclaimed through the door, "No! I can do it ALL MY BYSELF!" That story would be told and retold every time we went back to that store.

She didn't only shop for children's clothes. She was known to buy the nicest dresses and shoes at local department stores like Goudchaux's and D.H. Holmes, as well as small boutiques like R.F.D., Carriage's, and later, Harold's. Her favorite dress shop was called Bernie's and I think she enjoyed talking with all the other ladies in the store as much as she enjoyed buying clothes.

Bernie's had a particular scent. I'm not sure what it was, but whenever my mom would give new clothes to me or my sisters, we could immediately tell if it was from Bernie's just by the smell of the box before we even opened it. All four of her girls were set throughout high school and college with complete wardrobes of fine outfits and shoes.

Later, when Peggy lived in Tyler, Texas and then Dallas, my mom would take me to visit her and we would go on enormous shopping sprees. There were so many stores that we didn't have in Baton Rouge, so we could find stylish, unique clothes that no one else back home would be wearing. I was in awe when I first saw the Galleria and North Park Mall. I was thrilled to go through Neiman Marcus, Bloomingdale's, Saks Fifth Avenue, Macy's, Marshall Fields, and many others. We would come home with wardrobes of dresses, skirts, blouses, and shoes. We continued to travel to Dallas to buy clothes through my college years. I recently reread a letter my mom sent to me when I was a freshman in college. Among other valuable advice, she wrote, "Never go without something essential because of a lack of funds, and a new dress is essential!"

One of Mildred's most important rituals of self-care was her Thursday morning hair appointment at Pace's. She went to Janice Pace every week for most of her adult life. Each week, her hair was carefully washed, rolled, dried, teased, brushed, and sprayed into a coif that would last her until the next Thursday morning. Occasionally, she would have it cut and permed, which would cause the appointment to last longer. She never had her hair colored, though. By the time I came around she already had curls of salt, pepper, and silver hair. The only way I know she was brunette is from old photographs or slides taken of her before I was born.

If school was out for vacation or summer and there was no one to sit with me, I was required to attend this ritual. Pace's was a fascinating place for me. Its classic 1960s décor was unbeatable. Upon entering, we had to walk through strings of wooden beads in bright colors of orange, lime green, blue, and yellow. These strings of beads were also used to separate the different areas of the beauty parlor—and that's what it was—not a salon! Pace's was a beauty parlor.

Immediately upon entering, I was overcome by the scents of shampoo, nail polish remover, permanent solution, and, of course, Aquanet hairspray. I would wander around the rooms, twirling in the round, bowl-shaped orange chairs in the waiting area, or just sit under a dryer studying the different colors of nail polish. Meanwhile, my mother would soak in her weekly supply of gossip while getting her hair "done" for the week. That's what she did. Every Thursday morning, she went to Pace's to get her hair "done." And this element of her schedule was absolutely non-negotiable.

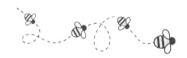

The age gap in my family not only meant I spent more time with my parents, but I was also a bit spoiled. There. I said it. I admit it. The other siblings knew it the whole time and I'm not sure how they felt about it, but it's true. Accordingly, unlike the others who had to share attention with four other siblings, I spent much of my youth living like an only child. It was not just being alone, but also the fact that my parents had spent over thirty years raising children and were kind of over it when it came to me. I was the only girl who had a short haircut for most of my childhood, and I have to think this is because my mom was just done fixing braids and pigtails by the time I came along. (Of course, I got these haircuts at Pace's—usually propped up on a booster seat). I was also allowed to drive earlier than my brothers and sisters. I'm sure this was because they were tired of driving to and from after school activities and practices, orthodontist appointments, sleepovers with friends, and everywhere else teens have to be taken.

While I was spoiled by being the youngest and probably spent more time with my parents while I was younger, the age gap had a major drawback. From as early as I can remember, I knew that I would lose them. This became one of my biggest fears, although I kept this a secret. I would sometimes calculate how old they would be when I became 20, 25, 30, etc. and try to guess if this was a reasonable age to expect them to live. It sounds morbid, and maybe by thinking about it and fearing it, I manifested it. It eventually came true, and I suffered great loss at young ages when most people couldn't imagine going through such things.

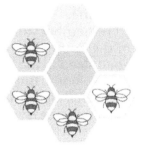

9

Not only did the age gap cause my sisters and me to have different types of relationships with my parents, it also meant we had completely different experiences with my grandmother. It's already been said that Mildred did not have the most affectionate relationship with her mother, especially after her dad was killed. But my grandmother was kind and loving to all her grandchildren, and I believe Mildred welcomed that, especially since it meant free babysitting for the children when she did manage to get Red away from his drawing table. She made frequent trips to Baton Rouge to stay with us and was always a welcome sight at Christmas and other holidays.

I'm not sure what my first memory is of my grandmother. My earliest memories are of going to Lake Charles to stay at her apartment, and of her coming to Baton Rouge to stay with us. I always looked forward to these visits. She would take Jane and me to the Pack-a-Sack or TG&Y and buy us the *Teen Beat* magazines, Fun Dip candy, and other things that my mom always said "no" to. Isn't that what grandmothers do? They spoil their grandkids. Say "yes" when mom said "no." And teach. Teach beautiful lessons about growing up and life.

My older siblings have different memories of MawMaw Wallace. (We pronounced it Maw Maw, but I always spelled it Mama; however, to avoid confusion, I will spell it MawMaw for this story). She lived in Kinder, Louisiana where she raised my mom and her three younger siblings. My older sisters remember visiting her house there. I remember stories of a large porch that wrapped around most of the house. This is where my mom and aunt and uncles would go to sleep in the hot Louisiana summers before air conditioning came along. But these are just stories to me. I don't think I've even seen a picture of the house, but I have the picture in my head. I can imagine trying to fall asleep, sweaty, swatting at mosquitoes, and waiting for a slight breeze to cool me off. I can imagine waking up early to birds chirping, morning dew on everything from the thick humid air cooling in the night. And maybe even a slight chill, at least compared to the evening before.

By the time I came along, MawMaw already lived in an apartment in Lake Charles. It was closer to my Aunt Bertie's house, so she had family nearby, but not so far away from Kinder as Baton Rouge or Houston, where my uncle lived. While my older sisters were away at camp (except Peggy, who was already married—she never got to go to camp, and we continue to hear about that to this day), my mom would drive me to Lake Charles to spend at least two weeks. I guess she and my dad needed a break from six kids every now and then. At the time, I just thought of it as the camp you go to until you are old enough for real summer camp.

During those weeks, I would go back and forth between staying at my aunt's house and my grandmother's apartment. Given a choice, I would have chosen MawMaw's apartment. For starters, my aunt's house was constantly filled with cigarette smoke. She chain smoked, despite my uncle's asthma. No windows open, and the house was small. You couldn't get away from it as long as you were inside. The other thing was the scary dog. Now, she was a tiny dog, a Chihuahua. But she wasn't like Bruiser from *Legally Blond*. Her name was Dixie, and she was mean. From the minute I woke up in my cousin's bed, she would be growling and baring her teeth at me. She seemed poised and ready to attack as soon as I made a wrong move. I was constantly afraid of this dog. But, I was definitely more afraid of complaining—about the smoke or the dog. Aunt Bertie's favorite phrase was, "I'll give you something to cry about!" In her deep husky voice, this phrase was scarier than any growl Dixie could muster up. So, my memories of staying at Aunt Bertie's house mostly consist of fear.

My grandmother's apartment, on the other hand, was heaven to me. She had an avocado green vinyl sofa that folded out into a bed! In the early 1970s, this was something so novel to me. It was always an adventure to fold out the couch and put the sheets and covers on it to get ready for a whole night of sleeping in the living room. Now that was special. She also made the absolute best chocolate chip cookies. I think that's also something grandmothers do. I bet if you asked my nieces and nephews, they would say that my mom made the best chocolate chip cookies. For some reason, a grandmother's cookies are always better than a mother's.

Not only did I get a sofa bed in the living room and cookies, but MawMaw's apartment had a pool! I could swim as much as I wanted, provided an adult was watching me. This consisted of my swimming alone all day with my grandmother sitting in a chair by the side of the pool. I never saw her swim, and today question her ability to do anything to save a drowning child other than call 911, but she watched and I swam.

MawMaw loved to sit on the sofa with me and show me old photo albums. All the pictures were black-and-white. I didn't recognize anyone in the photos, but she would carefully point out who everyone was and tell stories about them. I don't really remember the stories or the people in the photos. I just remember sitting close to her and hearing them. She seemed to have happy memories and to be content with her life. I was always comfortable around her and felt her to be a sincerely loving and generous lady.

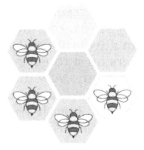

10

I WAS IN JUNIOR high when MawMaw started to forget things. She would tell the same stories over and over again. Sometimes she wouldn't remember what we were planning to do the next day or what we had done the previous day. She still recognized all her loved ones, made visits to Baton Rouge, and participated in family activities. But we knew things were changing. And I know my mom did not like it.

The summer after I finished the eighth grade, Jane got married. I was not thrilled about this because I felt like I was losing her permanently and I believe I was jealous of her soon-to-be husband for getting more time with her than I did. Remember, I was the pest that followed her around and idolized her. This was also the summer that Jane got more attention than I did. There were announcement parties, several showers, a bridesmaid luncheon, the rehearsal and rehearsal dinner, and the wedding and reception. And of course, for all these events, Mildred made sure that her daughters had the finest new dresses.

Jane's wedding was large. I mean, at least twelve bridesmaids. All dressed in puffy taffeta dresses. It would have been "Blush and Bashful" like Shelby's wedding in *Steel Magnolias*, but Goudchaux's got the order mixed up, and when the bridesmaids dresses came in they were lavender. There was no time to have them all remade, so Jane settled for the light purple wedding. At least the flowers still somewhat matched. Also, Peggy was able to get some of the lavender fabric in time to have Charlotte's flower girl dress made to match the rest of the wedding party.

I was excited when the actual wedding day arrived. The only thing that kept it from being perfect for me was that my brother Jack, who was supposed to be my escort down the aisle, backed out at the last minute (he was very shy and uncomfortable with any attention). Therefore, I had to walk down the aisle with Bill. Bill had already hogged the bathroom that morning from Jane—ahem, the BRIDE, and nearly hit her while kicking a drawer shut in his fit of anger. But other than that short procession out of the church, I was thrilled the whole day.

The wedding reception was held at my parents' house. As I mentioned earlier, my mom was famous for hosting large parties and the house was built for entertaining. The furniture had been rearranged to accommodate the crowd and the home was adorned with flowers and beautifully decorated. Red had worked countless hours outside to have the yard in perfect shape for an August wedding. Aunt Bertie, who was a school teacher but catered and decorated custom cakes on the side, had made and decorated an enormous cake with flowers that matched the fluffy taffeta dresses. Beer and champagne were served in the cleaned and decorated carport—only punch was served inside, and it was not spiked.

During all this excitement, I saw my grandmother sitting alone on one of the long white vinyl couches in the family room. I could've used a break from the party, so I took a seat next to her to relax. As we sat together, a group of bridesmaids walked past us towards the sliding glass door to go outside. As they walked by, MawMaw turned to me and asked, "Virginia, why in the world are all those girls wearing the same dress?"

I was baffled by this question and responded, "MawMaw, those are bridesmaids from Jane's wedding! Look, I'm wearing the same dress too!"

She looked at me confused and asked, "Oh, Jane got married? When?"

I stated, "MawMaw, we just came from the wedding. This is the reception. Don't you remember?"

She did not remember. And that's when I became aware of Alzheimer's for the first time, a disease that would haunt our family for years to come. Alzheimer's is a devastating illness for both the patient and their loved ones. It is so painful to watch someone you care deeply about lose their memory and then later, their personality. It requires children to become caregivers while losing the one who most cared for them. It has been described to me as a living death. I would not know it as that until much later in my life. But there, at Jane's wedding, on the couch with MawMaw, I also became aware that unless you can find some humor in a situation over which you have no control, you cannot survive it.

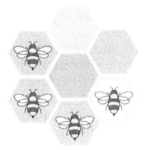

11

MawMaw's disease progressed slowly, but she was changed forever. She could no longer drive us to the store to buy treats. She could not travel to Baton Rouge on her own to visit. She couldn't babysit, although by then, even the youngest of her grandchildren did not require a babysitter. She also had become incontinent, which made her have the odor of stale urine rather than her usual soap or perfume.

I could tell my mom was saddened by the change, but she expressed it as a mixture of frustration and anger. She would fuss at her mother for forgetting things and ask her why she couldn't just remember this or do that. We all knew that what MawMaw had was bad and would not improve. But instead of grieving, we began to tell the stories of the things she did or said and laugh. And sometimes we would begin belly laughing to the point where tears came down our cheeks. The tears from laughter felt so much better than the tears that come when you let yourself feel the loss.

Instead of the nice, thoughtful gifts she usually sent us for birthdays and Christmas, Mawmaw had begun regifting household items from around her home. Her gift wrapping style certainly became unique as well. In fact, at Jane's wedding, sitting on the table among the beautifully wrapped white, silver, and gold wedding gifts, was MawMaw's wedding gift for Jane. But her gift was resourcefully wrapped in aluminum foil rather than paper and held together with Band-aids instead of tape! Yes, that day we knew something was wrong.

After a while, my mom and her siblings agreed that it was no longer safe for MawMaw to live alone in her apartment. While Aunt Bertie lived in Lake Charles close to MawMaw and Kinder, it made more sense to them for her to live with my Uncle Hubert in Houston. Aunt Bertie had health issues of her own and Hubert (or Bennie—his first name) had a larger home with a guest apartment that could accommodate MawMaw while still allowing her some independence.

They gathered together in Lake Charles to go through MawMaw's things, move what they could to Houston, and clean out the rest of her apartment. While cleaning out the kitchen, they discovered over twenty opened jars of mayonnaise in her refrigerator! I'm not sure what she was planning to do with them. I guess she just kept forgetting she already had mayonnaise every time she went to the store. But mayonnaise was just the beginning of the accumulation of junk that needed to be disposed of before her move to Houston.

Once she was settled into Uncle Hubert's guest house, MawMaw did not improve, but her dementia seemed to taper and things were not looking as bleak as they had been. Then one Sunday morning, MawMaw woke and dressed up for a morning with Hubert and his family. They attended Sunday school and church, then all went out to Sunday dinner at a nice restaurant. Upon returning home, Hubert changed and settled in a chair in his living room to watch football. During the game he was startled when MawMaw marched into the room right up to him and exclaimed, "Well, I'm not dead yet!"

"Well, Mother, I'm glad to hear that. Is there something wrong?" Hubert replied, confused.

"I've been sitting out in that apartment alone for an entire week and no one has even once bothered to check on me!" MawMaw answered in anger, just as sure of herself as can be.

"You've got to be kidding me. We just spent the entire morning together. You mean to tell me you do not remember going to Sunday school, church, or even lunch?"

"I did no such thing. I haven't left that apartment for over a week and you have left me all alone!"

For Hubert, this was the last straw. Hubert, Charlie, Bertie, and Mildred made the decision that it was time for MawMaw to go to a nursing home. Once again, her things were packed and she was settled into a facility in Lake Charles, central to where all the siblings could drive to visit her within a day.

What's so sad for me is that I do not remember the last time I saw MawMaw. We had denied her condition as an illness and instead just laughed, telling stories of the seemingly ridiculous things she had been saying and doing. While my mother visited her, she did not want me to see her in that place or see how her disease was progressing. Therefore, she never took me to visit MawMaw in the nursing home. Whatever my mother experienced there must have been so bad that she by no means wanted any of her children to go through the same thing. The rest of her life, every now and then, she would repeatedly and resolutely tell us, "If I EVER get to be like that, I want you to immediately lock me up in a nursing home and FORGET ABOUT ME! I'm serious. Do not ever visit me. Just leave me there and forget about me." This wish of hers would come back to me years later and continually haunt me.

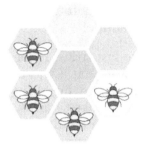

12

GROWING UP, KATHERINE, JANE, and I had spent our summers going to Camp Sequoya in Abingdon, Virginia. It was a beautiful place set in the mountains, and we spent a glorious four weeks away from the Louisiana heat, meeting new friends and learning how to water ski, sail, canoe, and do all sorts of other activities. Katherine and Jane had already been going while I was still spending summers between Aunt Bertie's and MawMaw's in Lake Charles. Once I turned eight years old, I was allowed to go. The summer after second grade was my first of fourteen summers at camp.

When I was a junior in high school, Katherine was working in Colorado, where she had held several different positions at Keystone Ski Resort. During that year, the director of Camp Sequoya contacted Katherine to offer her a position as Assistant Director at camp. Since the ski area was closed in the summers, Katherine had held a variety of summer jobs during her years at Keystone. She welcomed the opportunity to do something different and get to experience camp again. Therefore, my last year as a CIT (Counselor in Training), I was once again at camp with my sister.

As I said, growing up, I followed Jane around and wanted to be just like her. She was my only playmate at home, which made her the sister I was closest to. Now that I was seventeen, Jane was the busy mother of her first daughter, Elizabeth. While I loved Jane and adored Elizabeth, the life of being a mom was foreign to me. Meanwhile, Katherine was back at camp and getting to know my friends. We grew closer and began to have much more in common than before.

While I wanted to follow in Jane's footsteps as a young child, I began to follow Katherine. One thing Katherine had done that was borderline sacrilegious in our family was to attend the University of Alabama. Not only had my parents both gone to LSU, they also had served as President of the Alumni Association, on the Athletic Council, on the LSU Union Governing Board, and hosted every reunion for the LSU Class of 1942. My dad did not miss an LSU home football game in almost fifty years. Going to Alabama was to go against everything they stood for. But my parents were proud of Katherine and put such a value on education that they were happy to send her.

After that summer at camp with Katherine, I was back in Baton Rouge and ready for my senior year in high school. My siblings and I had all gone to LSU Lab School, which is a K-12 school located on the LSU campus and formed by the LSU Department of Education as a place to send student teachers to learn and practice methods before graduation. I only went there for 11th and 12th grade, but my friends there were as close to me as any other friends I had growing up. During our senior year, three of my best friends had decided to go to Alabama for college. Since I had been in high school on the LSU campus, I figured I'd try going away, so I headed to University of Alabama—just like Katherine.

Alabama was different from LSU, but fun. I pledged Chi Omega sorority and made many new friends while also staying close to the other Baton Rouge girls from my high school. My roommate Kim and I had many adventures in the dorm, especially playing pranks on the RA (Resident Assistant) assigned to our floor. Someone had told us that we could slide pennies in the small gap between the door and the door jamb to prevent it from opening. We tried it on her door and soon received a call.

"I need help! Somebody coined me in my room!" she exclaimed over the phone.

"What? What does that even mean?"

"I've been coined in my room, I can't get out."

"I don't understand. How do you get coined in your room?"

We went back and forth with her trying to control our laughter until we finally walked down the hall and somehow fished the coins from the door jamb and freed the RA.

I think I had a little too much fun my freshman year at Alabama because I made the worst grades I had ever made. I was an above average student most of my life, but with the freedom college dorm life gave me and the constant parties going on, school was not one of my priorities that year. Every Thursday night there was some kind of sorority/fraternity "swap" party, which didn't help my grades on the chemistry quizzes my professor gave at 8 every Friday morning. I wasn't a great student, but I learned the fight song, went to every home football game, and experienced all of the social events that went along with attending the University of Alabama. When the semester was coming to a close, I realized I was going to have to really cram in order to pass most of my courses.

In December of my freshman year, I was preparing for final exams when I got the call. MawMaw had passed away. My mom did not want me to miss my finals to attend her funeral. I guess it had been so long since I had seen her and she had been sick for so long, that hearing of MawMaw's death wasn't surprising or devastating to me. I agreed to do as my mom asked and stay at school. She had already spoken to Kim's parents, and they had agreed to drive me home to Baton Rouge for the Christmas holidays. I guess that was my first taste of homesickness while I was at Alabama.

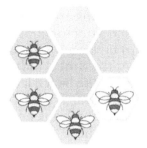

13

By now, Katherine had accepted a year-round position as Assistant Director of Camp Sequoya and had moved from Colorado to Bristol, Virginia. During the spring semester, I visited Katherine in Bristol. One of my Alabama sorority sisters was from the area, and I rode home with her for Easter. Even though I was in college and Katherine was in her thirties, we received a package from my mom. Inside were two Easter baskets, complete with stuffed bunnies, chocolate candy, and clothes which, from the smell, obviously came from Bernie's. Like I said, Mildred never skimped on a holiday.

The summer after my freshman year, I was back at camp as a counselor. There were two sessions of camp, each four weeks long. Since I was eight, I had only attended first session. As a counselor, I always planned on staying for second session. I mean, we were outside, doing fun activities with friends we don't see all year, and getting paid for it! Most of my friends stayed the whole summer. However, in each of my four years as a counselor, something always made me want to go home after first session. It was this odd homesick feeling. Something inside me needed to be near my parents and in Baton Rouge.

I went back to Alabama for the first semester of my sophomore year. This time I lived in an apartment with three other girls. We loved the freedom from the dorm and had so much fun together in that place. Then, once again, I got "the call." My dad had to have a mole removed from his arm. He had been ignoring my mom's pleas for him to see a doctor about it (not wanting to miss work), but when it got to be larger than a silver dollar, he finally went. It was melanoma. At the time, I didn't know anything about skin cancer. I still laid out on the beach lathered in baby oil trying to get my freckled skin as tan as it could be. We didn't have the internet, and I didn't have any books or magazines about it. I refused to believe it was anything bad.

My mom explained that he would be having a procedure during which surgeons would remove the mole and take skin from his upper thigh and graft it onto his arm. Then the oncologists would perform a type of chemotherapy that would go in through an artery in his upper arm, travel throughout that arm, and come out through a vein in the same arm. The chemotherapy would not enter the rest of his body. He would not lose his red hair! In fact, my dad joked about it. The procedure would have to take place at the Tulane Medical Center in New Orleans. He said he was going there to donate blood before so that, if something went wrong and he needed a transfusion, they wouldn't give him any green blood!

I felt relief. Well, it *was* cancer. A word I had always feared. But I thought it must not be a big deal because it was just moving some skin and he didn't even have to lose his hair. I thought the only people who could die of cancer were the ones who had the real chemotherapy and lost all their hair. Now, I know this was naïve, but it was 1988 and I was 19 years old. And I wanted to believe that it wasn't bad. Besides, he couldn't die. I had done the calculations. *When I'm 30, he'll be 80, but he's really healthy, so he'll live to be 90, which means I don't have to worry about things like this until I'm at least 40. Whew!* I had it all figured out in my head.

Even though I didn't take the news of the melanoma too seriously, it had to be what finally figured into my decision to leave Alabama and transfer to LSU. I had been filled with that same homesick feeling that kept me from staying for the second session of camp. I needed to be near my parents for some reason. That fall, after my dad's procedure, my parents traveled to Tuscaloosa for the Alabama v. LSU football game. Katherine also drove down for it. I met up with all of them before the game, dressed in a purple outfit, but carrying a red and white shaker. LSU beat Alabama that year, and when I saw my family after the game, I reached up my sleeve and pulled out a purple and gold shaker, having discarded the red and white one. That's when I announced that I was coming home to be a Tiger.

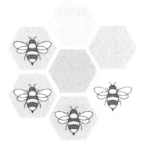

14

MY DECISION TO GO to LSU turned out to be the right one. Not only did my grades improve, but I had a great time as well. I spent these years in different apartments with different roommates, a semester in the Chi Omega sorority house, and some time living at home. I went to class...well, most of the time. I frequently spent my evenings at college bars like Murphy's, Fred's, the Dugout, and more that I don't even remember. I saw friends from high school and met new friends from all over the state. I was home, but I wasn't staying at home. I visited my parents, but I wasn't controlled by them. Also, Jane was living in Baton Rouge, so I could visit with her and spend time with my nieces, Elizabeth and Brittany. And I loved the LSU atmosphere—especially the football games.

I had been going to LSU football games for as long as I could remember. My parents had season tickets and their seats were surrounded by several of their friends. The seats next to theirs belonged to a couple that were close friends with my parents. When the husband died, his widow rode with my parents to all of the games and they began to bring me along with the spare ticket. We always had to be in the stadium while the team was still warming up and we stayed until the game was over. The score could be 70-3 and the weather freezing rain, but my dad's response to any request to leave early was, "The opera's not over until the fat lady sings."

I'm not sure there's a better place on Earth to be on a Saturday night in the fall than in Tiger Stadium. LSU fans are some of the loudest in the nation and take their football seriously. The band has a different song for every down and the entire crowd cheers along. Most would agree that the best part of the band is the pre-game show. When they march onto the field and blast those first four notes and the crowd erupts, I still get chills all over my body. To this day I love the sights, sounds, smells, and feel of college game day in Baton Rouge. Whether LSU is winning or losing, the experience is a unique one that everyone should experience. Now I understand why my dad's home game attendance streak was so important to him.

I was a junior at LSU when the C word reared its ugly head again. We found out my mom had breast cancer. Once again, I was told it was not bad. It had been caught early. The tumor was the size of a pea. She had a lumpectomy followed by radiation. It was strange but sweet to see my dad take over the caregiving role. He was with her at every radiation appointment. It was obvious he was worried about her and wanted her to have the best treatment and to survive.

After the radiation, my mom was placed on a drug called tamoxifen. This was the new miracle cure for breast cancer. She would not need any more radiation and no chemotherapy, as long as she stayed on this medicine. The whole family breathed a sigh of relief. We knew we could not go on without my mom. She was the glue that held us all together. The oil that kept the machinery working. Without her, what would my dad do? What would any of us do? Hence, the favorable diagnosis was welcome.

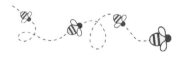

I was not the only one moving in and out of my parents' house during this time. Throughout my high school and college years, my brothers Bill and Jack spent time living there as well. Bill had been divorced and returned to LSU to earn a Ph.D. in computer science. This feat ended up taking him eight years. Although my parents eventually forced him out and into an apartment, he would invariably be found at their house. Usually, he showed up just in time for dinner. Other times, he would just spend long afternoons lounging in front of their TV, eating huge bowls of ice cream with his tight T-shirt tucked all the way into his high-waisted sweatpants.

Jack, on the other hand, lived with my parents for a different reason. After high school, he spent his years working on tugboats along the Mississippi River. He also served in the United States Marine Corps. While he was stationed overseas in Guam, my parents received a letter from the Marine Corps doctor posted there. The doctor wrote that Jack had been sent to him for an examination and the doctor had reached a preliminary diagnosis of schizophrenia. Jack was transferred to a desk job until he was honorably discharged and sent home.

Jack was taken to the VA hospital in Gulfport, Mississippi. When he was discharged, he lived with my parents. He went back and forth between that hospital and their house for several years. My parents did not discuss Jack's condition with us, and I knew not to ask too many questions. I will admit it was awkward for me having him in the house while I was in high school, but that's because I was a self-absorbed teenager with no empathy for anyone else. Once I was in college, however, I enjoyed the time I spent with Jack.

I did not grow up living in the house with my brothers, so it was mainly during my high school and college years that I got to know them. Jack was always quiet, but quick to help with anything that needed to be done. I can remember him and my dad splitting wood in the backyard for hours on weekends so that our fireplace could be consistently lit during the winter. I also remember Bill in front of the TV, eating ice cream while they were working outside. He seldom lifted a finger to help anyone, but he was quick to take firewood to give to his friends.

I will give Bill credit for the one good thing I remember him doing for me. He taught me how to drive a stick shift. I remember he had an old Porsche 924. It had once been silver, but by then it looked rusted and old. He was the type who would rather have a bad Porsche than a good Chevrolet. But that's beside the point. Teaching me to drive that Porsche required a tremendous amount of patience. I remember being stopped at a red light on an uphill road. I was so scared of pulling my foot off the clutch and rolling into the car behind us that I made him get out and go ask the driver if he would back up and give me a little more space. I later owned a Jeep with standard transmission, and I owe Bill for being able to drive such a great car.

When it came to family time, most of it centered around the kitchen table. My mom prepared a hefty breakfast every morning and a full course dinner every night. We would sit around the table eating her roast and rice and gravy, fried chicken, pork chops, spaghetti, and many other Mildred specialties. Usually, the conversation would last longer than the dinner, and we would all linger in the kitchen. I enjoyed hearing my dad tell stories. He had great jokes—they were corny dad jokes, but I loved them. Whether he discussed his work, LSU, memories of the war in Europe, or any other topic, I would listen. Jack was always quiet, but he stayed at the table and took in the conversation. Occasionally he might even offer an insight of his own.

When Bill was at the table, it was a different kind of mealtime. He launched into diatribes about his dissertation and computers, geological surveys, his supervisor at LSU, and any other topic. I mean ANY other topic. I used to joke that if I started talking about my last period, I'm sure Bill would chime in and know more about it than I did! My parents listened patiently and tried not to interrupt, but I could feel the pull to get away from the table from every direction.

It was just common knowledge to all of us that Bill was obnoxious. I mean, we even couldn't stand the way he sneezed! He would blast out the loudest nasal explosion while his voice seemed to yell out something which sounded like "AHH-CHAW!" and we either cringed or stifled a laugh until we could all be alone together and cackle about it, repeating to each other: "AHH AHH AHH-CHAW!"

In college, I enjoyed conversations with Jack. He liked to watch the news and he often discussed politics with me. We also did some running together. I had run cross country in high school and was then trying to keep it up just to stay in shape. As we ran around the neighborhood, he would chant like a Marine and I would follow along, "Hoo-rah! Feels Good!" with every other step. I wanted to do more with him and I always had ideas of activities I thought we would enjoy together. I often thought of taking him to a bar I liked called Uncle Earl's to play pool together, now that I was legally old enough. Then I would put my ideas to the side so that I could enjoy my college social life and my friends. After all, I could always spend time with him later.

15

I WAS ASLEEP IN my pull-out bed on the second floor of the Chi O house on March 15, 1990. I was hung over from some kind of party the night before, and had already skipped several classes, when the phone rang. I reluctantly answered it, aggravated at having been awakened. The first words Jane said to me were, "Jack's dead."

"What?"

"Jack died. He killed himself. I'm coming to pick you up. You need to get ready."

"What?"

"I'll be there in a little while. Just get dressed and I'll fill you in when I get there."

I hung up the phone in shock! This couldn't be true. Could I go back to sleep and wake up from this bad dream? Reality slowly began to sink in. My body began to tremble and my chest tightened. That's when I started sobbing—loud, uncontrollable sobs that could be heard by everyone in the hall. Immediately, girls were surrounding me and trying to find out what happened and comfort me. All I could say was, "My brother's dead." Some

girls hugged me tightly while I sobbed. I'm not even sure who
was there. I eventually broke away and made it to my room to
get dressed. This was bad. Really bad. And I dreaded the rest that
was to come.

Jane got to the Chi O house shortly and I climbed into her van.
We hugged and cried and then proceeded to drive to my parents'
house. On the way, she filled me in as much as she could about
what had happened. Jack had been found dead from a type of
overdose in a hotel off the interstate in Baton Rouge. The police
came to the house to notify my parents. Bill was the only one
there and immediately called for our pastor, George Haile, to
meet my parents at the house. (He was always the first person
to arrive at the hospital or home to offer care and support when
any of us needed it.) While my parents were hearing the news,
Jane had driven up with Elizabeth and Brittany for a visit. Once
she figured out what had happened, she had maintained her
composure for the sake of her girls, brought them to a sitter, and
called me. Now we were in the driveway and knew we had to go
inside, no matter how desperate I was not to face this reality.

The next moment and days blur together in my memory.
George Haile greeted me and hugged me tightly in an effort to
console me. I remember that my dad had to go identify the body.
I remember my mom's tears as she tried to muster the strength
to face planning a funeral as well as speak to the seemingly
endless stream of friends and relatives visiting the house to offer
condolences. The funeral would be soon, but we would need to
wait for Peggy and Katherine to come into town in time for the
services.

The evening that we found out, I climbed into the bed next to
my mother and snuggled her. My dad wasn't in the room yet. I
didn't remember too much Shakespeare from high school, but
this one nugget was stuck in my head.

"Did Jack read any Shakespeare, Mom?" I asked.

"I'm not sure, why do you ask?"

"Because of that famous quote from Julius Caesar, 'Beware the
Ides of March.' Do you think he chose this day to die because it's
the Ides of March?"

She didn't have an answer for me. Nothing made sense to any of
us.

The other memory that stands out to me will stay ingrained in my memory as a sort of nightmare forever. I have never liked to see a grown man cry. I am very sentimental and cry at a Hallmark commercial, so the sight of a grown man crying is just the saddest thing to me. Now, make that grown man my father, Red Evans, strong, smart, honest, hardworking, and ever faithful. The following day, I accidentally walked into my parents' bedroom, where I know he thought he was alone. I saw my dad on his hands and knees, rocking back and forth, sobbing. I stepped out and ran to my bed to cover my face as I broke down. Since that day, I have learned a great deal more about mental illness and suicide. However, at that moment, all I could feel was anger towards Jack for making my dad hurt so much.

The next few days went by in a flurry. Friends and family in and out of the house, bringing all sorts of food. Going to the funeral home. Seeing Jack's face in the casket. They parted his hair in the middle. He always parted it on the side. How could they make such a mistake? Peggy hugging and comforting me in the car ride from the funeral home to the cemetery. Going back to the house and feeling numb and exhausted while people remained seemingly forever. Just wanting to go back in time and this not to have happened. But it did happen. And our family was forever changed.

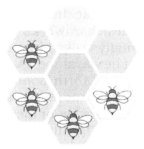

16

IF MILDRED AND RED Evans were anything, they were resilient. I've always heard that there is no greater pain than the loss of a child. Though they continued to mourn, they got back to their routines of going to the office, PEO and Kiwanis meetings, church, and social events. When something bad happens to me, I usually curl up into a ball and shut down in a fit of depression. Not them. I guess that's the difference between The Greatest Generation and a spoiled Gen Xer like me. Not that I haven't survived tough times, but I've never done it with my parents' style of strength and dignity.

That spring of my junior year, I eventually went back to the sorority house for the rest of the semester. I attended parties and still managed to make decent grades. My friends were an incredible source of strength for me. They were always there for me if I needed to talk, or if I just needed to go out and have a good time and not think about anything. Once school was out, I was off to camp again and was more than excited to get away. While I had a great time and enjoyed being with Katherine and my friends, I once again left for home after the first session. That homesickness for my parents and for Baton Rouge stung me again.

I thoroughly enjoyed my senior year at LSU. I had no idea what I was going to do after college and I had changed my major course of study several times. One aching need I had most of my life was the need to please my parents. I did not ever want them to think I was a failure and I had a deep need to do the right thing in order to make them proud of me. The first wrong decision I made in this effort was to start off as a civil engineering major. While I could get Bs in math and science and could think logically, I couldn't draw a circle. I did not end up with the creative gene and was not talented in most any kind of art, especially drawing. After one semester of engineering graphics, attempting to draw machine parts to scale, I realized I would have to find another way to please them.

I ended up with a double major in history and economics and a minor in political science. I did not know what this kind of degree would qualify me to do in the future, but I wasn't concentrating on careers at that time. I lived with some friends in a duplex and we had some great parties. I even started my own tradition of decorating a tree like my mom. We had two kittens, who climbed and toppled it almost as soon as it was decorated. Eventually, we tied it to the wall somehow and kept it up through the Christmas season.

Over Mardi Gras break, I went on a snow skiing trip to Steamboat, Colorado with a group of friends. We drove straight through the night to Steamboat. We were following a group of boys in another car who refused to stop for a bathroom break, forcing me to strip and squat over an empty 44 oz. fountain drink cup and dump my pee out of the window! During Easter break, I went with a different group of friends to the beach in Hilton Head, South Carolina. Once again, we drove straight through the night and had a great time drinking and tanning on the beach. I guess something in me knew the real world was just around the corner, so I chose to enjoy the freedom of college as long as possible.

One of the first things that brought the reality of my age to me was being asked to be a bridesmaid in a friend's wedding. I had been to plenty of family weddings, but I was way too young to have friends who got married, right? I guess this reality check only encouraged my careless attitude. But it sure was fun and I wouldn't trade any of those good times for the world.

It was at the reception for the wedding in which I was a bridesmaid that I noticed my mom holding her side. She was standing next to my dad at the reception, wincing as she held one arm bent and close to her chest. I asked what was wrong and she just told me she had been having this ache in her side for a while. I looked at my father and back to her. I made her promise that she would see a doctor the next week if the pain did not go away. She agreed finally, and I returned to the reception.

The next week, we found out that the miracle breast cancer drug, tamoxifen, does not come without side effects. One such effect is that the drug can cause blood clots. And it had caused a blood clot to travel to one of my mother's lungs. She was immediately hospitalized for two weeks and put on an IV blood thinner called heparin. This treatment was meant to break up the clots in her body, including the one in her lung, while under the supervision of hospital doctors to ensure no more clots came loose and traveled to any other vital organs. Once she was discharged from the hospital, she was to remain on the blood thinning drug, Coumadin, until her five-year treatment with tamoxifen was finished. She was also supposed to wear compression hose and not remain seated too long at the office or traveling, but get up and walk around regularly.

As my mom recovered from the blood clot in her lung and became used to her regimen of Coumadin and regular blood tests to regulate the dosage, I returned to school and enjoying my senior year. When May came around, I had three courses left before I could graduate from LSU. I decided to finish these over the summer rather than go back to camp. I'm not sure why I was in a rush to graduate, because I still had not planned on what to do next. I suppose I felt like my parents had paid for enough and I should try to finish in as close to four years as possible for them.

Even with three courses, I managed to have a fun summer. I was able to visit Katherine and my friends at camp over a long weekend. I enjoyed time with my Baton Rouge friends. When August rolled around, I think my parents were proud to see their youngest child graduate from college. They were in their 70s after all, and getting through all six of their kids was quite an accomplishment. Or maybe they were just relieved. Anyway, they showed up beaming at the graduation ceremony. Afterwards, my family and friends gathered at my parents' house for a celebration with one of my favorite dishes that my mom made, boiled shrimp! I had been wanting a video camera and was elated to open my graduation gift and find one. Also, Jane made a wreath for me out of Styrofoam with crinkled $1 bills pinned all over it so it looked like leaves. It was tied with purple and gold ribbon. Imagine—an LSU money wreath. She always was, and still is, the most creative of the Four Bees.

Now it was time to decide what to do next. You can't exactly walk off of campus and do history. And I really had no idea what I wanted to do for a career. I enrolled in graduate school at LSU and took some classes in education and business. I figured I could get a taste of each and see if I might want to teach or go into business or public administration. Towards the end of 1991, I realized I wasn't interested in either. A friend of mine had recently moved to Dallas and started working for her aunt's mortgage company. She convinced me to go there and live with her for a while. So, after Christmas in 1991, I packed up my belongings and headed to Dallas to look for a job and start living on my own for the first time ever.

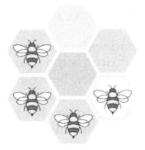

17

ARRIVING IN DALLAS, I was not prepared and was unclear as to what to expect. It was nothing like being in Tuscaloosa, Alabama or Bristol, Virginia. The highways were at least eight lanes wide and when getting on the interstate, you'd better be up to speed because there was no time to consider when you were going to merge. Even the side streets had up to six lanes. And the city was so vast. It seemed like it took at least thirty minutes to get from my apartment on Preston and Arapaho to anywhere. Also, I was expecting to see cowboy hats and boots everywhere. I was absolutely off on this count. Dallas was a fashion-forward city full of luxury automobiles and brand-named everything. It didn't take long for me to realize it took money to fit in here, and I didn't have any.

My first errand was to go to the bank and open a checking account. My friend, Molly, sent me to the bank where her uncles worked in downtown Dallas. The drive was an adventure in itself. I had no GPS or cell phone in 1992. I frequently had to stop to study my map and memorize my route before moving on. Once in the tall bank building, I was led to a desk off the lobby where I sat until Molly's uncle approached me. He tried to make conversation while I filled out the appropriate forms and deposited the money to open my account, order checks, and get an ATM card. I was so intimidated by the city, the size of the buildings, and the people that I could barely speak. I remember Molly telling me that her uncle called her at work to say, "You didn't tell me that your friend, Virginia, was so quiet and shy."

Molly almost spit up her coffee, "What?! Virginia is nothing like that. Are you sure it was her? I promise she is the opposite of quiet and shy. Just wait until you get to know her!"

When she called to ask me what had happened at the bank, I really didn't have an answer. To this day, I sometimes get this intimidating feeling in unfamiliar situations. At these times, my normally loud, outgoing personality disappears and I turn into someone quiet, shy, and seemingly unsure of herself. I hate it when I do that. It never works out well for me; whether it's a job interview or a client meeting, I have to fight my way out of it to try to even sound normal.

Eventually, Molly's aunts and uncles got to know the real me and I spent plenty of time with them. Getting to know one another over a few beers on their patio helped. They often cooked dinner for us, which was followed by stories outside by the pool while her uncle played his guitar and, occasionally, sang for us. Then, after a few weeks with no luck on my job hunt, one of her aunts offered me a job at the mortgage company where she served as president. I jumped at the opportunity because I needed to start earning some money. But I insisted that it was a temporary situation until I found my real job, whatever that meant.

I started working at Guardian Mortgage as a receptionist. I learned that the interest rates, which were then around 8%, were at an all-time low and everyone was seeking to refinance. Looking back, this seems outrageous. But at that time, people still had homes with mortgage interest rates in the teens and twenties, leftover from the Carter administration. The phone was constantly ringing, and I would take information from people seeking to buy or refinance their home and pass it along to loan officers, who would then set up appointments with the customers.

Within a few weeks, it was evident that I could catch on quickly to how things were done and the company might be able to use my skills elsewhere. I was moved to the payoff processing section. Here, I received checks to pay off the balance of a mortgage, usually because the borrower had sold or refinanced their home.

I was taught to calculate the balance as of the date the check was received and determine if the borrower was owed a refund, then continue the process of paying off the loan. The work was boring and at times it was hard to stay awake, even though we were extremely busy. But at least I had a job and a regular paycheck.

Soon I was moved to the closing department, where I remained for the rest of my time there. I prepared the documents which borrowers have to sign in order to secure the loan needed to purchase or refinance their home. The calculations and document understanding came easily to me, but it was more interesting than payoffs. And my desk was in the center of the floor, enabling me to interact with more people and even get to know the owner of the company. I was frequently telling jokes or acting ridiculous, always trying to get a laugh out of someone and break up the otherwise mundane day. The work was satisfying, and, with the low interest rates, I was often busy enough to clock in some overtime on the weekends.

Now that I was earning my own money, I began wanting to spend it. I had been spoiled and saving was not one of my priorities early on. The first thing I set my sights on was a Jeep Wrangler. Now, even though I planned on financing it and making all the payments myself, at 23, I still considered it important to ask my parents for their opinion. As usual, I approached my mom first. When she wanted the answer to be no, but she didn't want to be the one to say it, her answer to all of us was inevitably, "Ask your father." For my older siblings, this meant "no" and the conversation was over. I believe I was the only one who literally approached him and actually asked him for things. This wasn't the first time for me to overcome this hurdle, and I usually got the answer I wanted.

That evening I called and he answered the phone. I asked, "Dad, have you eaten dinner yet?"

"No, why?" he replied.

"No reason. I'll call you back in about an hour." Rule number one: make sure you ask when he has a full stomach.

One hour later I called back and he answered again. After some small talk, I started in, "Dad, I've been thinking, and well, the Pontiac Grand Am I'm driving is having a lot of problems. It's old, it has leaks, and it would be expensive to repair. I am working and have a salary now, so I would like to buy another car. Well, not just another car, I would like to buy a Jeep Wrangler."

Without hesitation he said, "Okay, that sounds like a good idea to me. I will sign the back of the title to the Grand Am and send it to you so you can trade it in. Maybe you should call the USAA car buying service. They can negotiate a price for you and provide financing for the new Jeep."

And that was it. I was going to buy a Jeep. I could almost feel my mother's blood boiling in the background. But she could have said no and ended it that afternoon. Instead, she chose the old "Ask your father" routine and it backfired on her. I don't believe she opposed the idea of my buying a car—I think she just believed Jeeps were dangerous and wanted me to have something safe and reliable instead.

I'll never forget the first time I drove that Jeep from Dallas to Baton Rouge for a visit. It was a hunter green color and, with the top down, I believe reminded my dad of the vehicles he had driven during his time in the army. He was so proud of me and that Jeep. He made me sit in it in the driveway and pretend to be driving while he took pictures of me. Then he brought a ladder out from the workshop, climbed up to the top step, and took more pictures of me from above. He wanted a view of me in that Jeep from every angle. It might not have been the most practical car I've ever owned, but it was fun to drive and worth watching the joy on my father's face every time he saw it.

One of the bonuses of moving to Dallas was that, for the first time in my life, I was living in the same place as Peggy. Technically, her home was in Allen, a town north of the city. But Dallas is sprawling and almost every residential area is a suburb, so I considered us as living in the same place.

I often visited her on the weekends. It was great to get home-cooked meals that reminded me of my mom. I would bring laundry up to her house and she would graciously help me wash, dry, and fold clothes while we ate and visited. While she couldn't spend money like my mom, she definitely inherited her shopping gene. Peggy knew where every mall was in the city and how to find anything you were looking for. She could shop for hours all over Dallas without buying a thing. Still does!

I also enjoyed getting to spend more time with my niece and nephew. Aaron was a senior in high school at the time. He and his friends sometimes visited my apartment. Besides his love for his grandparents, I believe I began to have an influence over him at this time, leading him to apply to LSU. I took him to crawfish boils and parties held by the Dallas chapter of the LSU Alumni Association. I also attended Charlotte's school plays. She was and is a talented actress with an avid love for theater.

When I was in Dallas, the Cowboys won two Super Bowls. Guardian Mortgage had several sets of season tickets to all sports events, but Cowboys tickets were in high demand and hard to come by. However, the owner of the company generously gave me tickets to see several of the Dallas Mavericks basketball games. The Mavericks were not exactly good at the time, but I enjoyed the games. It gave me a chance to spend more time with Peggy and her family, as I would invite them to come along. Even though the Dallas team wasn't playing well that year, we got to see legends like Michael Jordan, Charles Barkley, and Shaquille O'Neal (who I also had seen at LSU).

In the spring, I was able to convince my mom to visit us in Dallas for my birthday. I also tried to convince my dad to come, but he was too busy with work. I told him, "Now Dad, nobody ever said on their deathbed that they wish they had spent more time at the office."

"I know, but this project has to be done this week and there's no way around it. Next time."

Thus, my mom came alone. She, Peggy, and I shopped all over Dallas once again. While I did get a few things for my birthday, we made this trip about my mom. We took her to one of her favorite boutiques, St. John, where she bought knit dresses for parties, the office, meetings, and the LSU alumni center, along with casual pants and blouses for traveling and leisure time. She also bought shoes. I can't count the number of Ferragamo shoes that woman owned, but she sure added to the collection on that trip. She even got an orange pair just to match one of her new outfits. Remember, she was always well dressed and put together no matter what she was doing. I even have a picture of her on my refrigerator whitewater rafting in a matching St. John knit outfit!

Another 1992 milestone was that my dad moved his office from downtown Baton Rouge to the house. Since 1969, his home drawing room had always been unfinished. He carefully copied all our heights with the names and dates from the bare stud onto a paper he titled, "How High We Were." Sheetrock then covered the walls and the floor was carpeted. He was as busy as ever; however, now he was doing more work as an expert witness in legal matters involving faulty construction or design, especially roofing.

Later in 1992, Molly and I moved to a duplex closer to SMU. I liked the feel of being close to a university even though I wasn't going to school. I also missed the hours and freedom that came from attending school rather than a full-time job at a company. I started contemplating going back for some type of graduate degree, but I still didn't know what type. I stayed on at the mortgage company, enjoyed getting closer to Peggy and her family, and traveled home for more than one LSU football game. Overall, the year was a good one.

I believe I was meant to bond with Peggy that year in Dallas, just as I had bonded with Katherine while at camp, and Jane in Baton Rouge, because November 1992 was approaching and so was my parents' 50th wedding anniversary. I was in Dallas when I was informed of their plans for a family trip over Thanksgiving to Washington D.C. and Williamsburg rather than having a party to celebrate. I'm grateful to have had the opportunity to forge these bonds with each of my sisters before the trip and solidify our closeness for a lifetime.

18

After Thanksgiving, Peggy, Jane, and their families left Williamsburg on Saturday morning to head back to Dallas and Baton Rouge, respectively. That left Mom, Dad, Bill, Katherine, and me to spend the last day of the family vacation together. We relaxed and got in a little more sightseeing. All the while, Katherine spent her time calling the fine dining restaurants in the Colonial Williamsburg area for dinner reservations. That was one part of the plan Bill had neglected that had been bothering Katherine the whole trip. Sure enough, every single restaurant in the district required reservations well in advance and were completely booked. So much for an authentic colonial dining experience for the 50th wedding anniversary celebration.

I finally lost it.

When I finally stole my parents away from Bill for a few moments, I launched into it.

"You have let Bill plan this entire trip. He has only lived in Virginia for a few months, but you let him convince you he knows everything there is to know and dictate where everyone should be and when they should be there! The hotel and condominium choices were a disaster, the tour of the Archives was a nightmare, and now he has ruined the final night, the anniversary dinner?! And how do you think this made Katherine feel? She has spent nearly twenty summers in this state and lived here full-time for the better part of a decade. She has been to all the places you wanted to go and knew the areas and the best places to stay. But did you even bother to ask her opinion about one single thing? No! You just let Bill be the boss and make everyone else miserable in the process. I don't care about it as long as you enjoy your anniversary; however, you owe Katherine an apology and should show her some deference after what you've done!"

Well, I said it. I don't think I had ever spoken to my parents in that tone or with such criticism. My anger at Bill had just been building up for days and I couldn't stand by and let them keep treating him like the know-it-all he thought he was while ignoring the one of their children that actually could have given some good advice on how to plan this trip. I sat quietly and waited for my tongue-lashing. After all, I had already been chastised for staying out past midnight at my own sister's condo. This was much more disrespectful and surely deserved some blowback.

But my parents sat in silence. They didn't look angry. I might have even detected a glimpse of sadness in their faces, but it's hard to remember. All I know is for the rest of that day, before we went anywhere or did anything, my dad would say, "Well, Katherine, you've lived here longer than any of us and know more about the area. Why don't you suggest what we should do next?" They were trying a last-minute changing of the guard, replacing the boss of the trip. The problem was that it was already too late.

With no available restaurants in the historic area, we drove up and down the highway looking for an open place to eat dinner. I remember being curious about how many restaurants advertised that they had the best waffles and spaghetti in town. Did this mean they were great for breakfast and then turned into makeshift Olive Gardens at sunset? Or did people actually order these things together? (This was before chicken and waffles became a thing. But chicken and waffles make more sense together than waffles and Italian!) I declared I would not be eating at one of these establishments.

Then we saw it. Bob Evans Family Restaurant! I had never heard of it, but Katherine told me it was sort of like Cracker Barrel. Dad was already approaching the hangry point so there was no more time to be picky. And our last name was Evans, after all. As long as it wasn't named Bill Evans, I was okay with it.

So, there we sat. Eating family dinner bell plates with sweet tea. No candles, no champagne, no fancy tablecloths and menus. But, for that night, we all got along. And I think my dad probably enjoyed that meal more than he would have liked anything else. He was celebrating fifty years of marriage to Mildred Wallace Evans, the love of his life. And everything was golden.

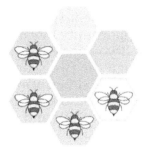

19

I RETURNED TO DALLAS as one of the Four Bees. Part of the group. I was now an adult and the age gap between my sisters and me seemed to have disintegrated. We had all hung out as friends. We went out together, shopped together, drank in the hot tub together, and joked and laughed as if there had never been any doubt that we would end up as a group. So what if Bill thought we were bitches? I wasn't exactly his biggest fan anyway. And now I had a group of sisters that were brought closer than ever by his ugly name-calling. I was happy with this new feeling of sisterhood and ready for whatever life chose to throw at me.

After the anniversary trip, I began to think seriously about going back to school for some kind of degree besides history. The owner of our company suggested law school. Hmmmm. I had never thought about that. Really. But I started to. After all, the closing documents I prepared were all sent to a lawyer's office to be signed. Lawyers didn't just chase ambulances and prosecute murderers. People needed a lawyer to buy a house. And buying a house was one of the biggest steps in one's life, up there with getting married or the birth of a child. I knew the industry. I started thinking seriously and studying for the LSAT.

In early 1993, I took the test for the first time. It was administered in Tyler, Texas. I had to wake up at 3 or 4 in the morning to get there in time. After the long drive, I got lost on the way to the testing facility. I was completely exhausted and flustered by the time I was handed the first exam booklet. At that time, the LSAT offered an opportunity to cancel your score prior to receiving your results. If you got your results and took the test over, they would average the two scores rather than use the highest. I was convinced I had performed horribly on the test in Tyler. I canceled the test without learning my score. I signed up for an LSAT prep class at SMU and started preparing more seriously. Later, I took the test at SMU, blocks from my duplex, much more prepared and calm. I don't remember my score; it wasn't outstanding, but it was above average.

I decided to apply to SMU law school. The owner of our company made me an extraordinary offer. He agreed to have the company pay for my law school tuition if I continued to work for them during and after law school. This was an opportunity I took very seriously and was beginning to see myself as a Dallas resident and lawyer. But that homesick part of me had a contingency plan and I also applied to law school at LSU.

While waiting to hear about my acceptance or rejection from law schools, Katherine and I made plans to travel to Hilton Head, South Carolina for a beach trip in May. The weekend before the trip was scheduled, we each had to make a short trip to Baton Rouge for the wedding of a friend from camp. It was a quick trip, with a flurry of activity and many friends to reunite and catch up with.

We stayed at my parents' house, but were busy with friends and wedding activities so we did not spend much time with them. I did notice that my dad didn't seem to be feeling well. He said he was getting over a cold and resting because he had a big jury trial coming up in which he was the star expert witness about some construction issues. Leaving for the airport, I hugged him goodbye. It was then I felt something in his upper abdomen, right below his ribcage, like a hard rock poking out of him. It didn't feel good, but I needed to get to the airport so I brushed the feeling aside and headed back to Dallas so I could pack and fly to Hilton Head.

Once in South Carolina, Katherine and I were perfectly relaxed. We had a great room with a screened-in porch overlooking the beach. We would spend hours in beach chairs, relaxing with drinks and music. We'd go out to dinners at some of the island's popular restaurants. Then repeat everything the next day. The subject only came up once, even though I know we both thought about it all week. I did not want to acknowledge it, as if saying it out loud would make it real and staying silent would make it go away. However, towards the end of the trip, while relaxing and drinking in our beach chairs, Katherine said it: "You know we're about to go through something really bad, right?"

"Yes, we are."

And that's all we said about it. We continued to enjoy our time off work, away from all our worries, and soak in the wonders of the ocean and sky.

20

UPON MY RETURN TO Dallas, I went with Molly to her aunt's house. We enjoyed drinks on her patio and her uncle played his guitar and serenaded us with his favorite songs. I was tan from the beach and relaxed from the trip. Not ready to go back to work but loving their company in their home. They had always treated me as one of the family and it felt good to be back there. Having her aunt as a friend and a boss was an interesting relationship, but was never awkward, and I was appreciative of all they had done for me since I had arrived in Dallas almost two years earlier.

A few nights later, Molly was at her boyfriend's apartment and I was alone in the duplex when the phone rang. It was my mom. My father's melanoma had returned. Apparently, it returned with a vengeance. It had metastasized, spreading throughout his body. He had not been feeling well and had finally gone to the doctor. After being dismissed twice with a diagnosis of arthritis, the doctor ran more tests on his third visit. They would be going to the oncologist the next day and would know more. I asked her to put my dad on the phone.

"Hi Dad," I began, "how are you feeling?"

"Oh, I'm okay, I guess. Except I can't seem to get these ABCs off the roof of my mouth."

What in the world was he talking about? I replied, "I'm going to fly to Baton Rouge to see you."

"You don't need to do that. I'm not sick. Everything is going to be fine."

I had him put Mom back on the phone and told her that I would be flying home the next day, then hung up.

This was it. I could feel it. My worst nightmare. I feared this moment for as long as I could remember. But I thought I had more time. I had done calculations. He was only 74. Plenty of people lived into their 80s and 90s. And he ate right. He exercised. No, this couldn't be happening. But I remembered that hug from a few weeks ago. That hard rock sticking out of his stomach. That was a lump. A tumor.

My chest felt tight. My heart was racing. My mind was all over the place. I couldn't think. My first call was to Molly's aunt to let her know that my father was sick, I was going to Baton Rouge, and I did not know when I would be back to work.

When my tears finally came, it was like a dam being opened. Once I started sobbing it seemed impossible to stop. "I'm too young to lose my dad!" I yelled to no one. "It's not fair!" Even though I feared this day forever, I wasn't prepared for it.

Somehow, I calmed myself down enough to call Southwest Airlines and book a flight to New Orleans for the next morning. (Remember, no internet.) Southwest was the least expensive, but it didn't fly into Baton Rouge. I don't remember calling my friends, but I must have because they were in New Orleans the next day to pick me up at the airport.

Then more sobbing. Everything was a blur. Either I called Molly or her aunt did. She showed up and we just sat. There wasn't much to say. I felt like my world was coming to an end. I hadn't even heard a prognosis yet, but I had given up. Now I just needed to get home, to Baton Rouge, to my parents.

I arrived at the New Orleans airport the next day. I actually saw some of my family there. Jane? Katherine? Mom? I don't remember. I just know I told them that I already had friends coming to pick me up and did not need a ride. I wasn't ready to see family yet. This wasn't real yet. Stay away. Make it go away.

Once I got home, I put on my brave face. I can do that when I have to. Really. I can push aside all the emotion and take care of the business at hand. I know this now. I have done it a million times, it seems. But, this must have been the first time. It was new for me. But I had to do it, so I did.

I hugged my dad. I felt the lump poking out of him. I asked him how he was feeling.

"Well, I'm okay. Except, now I know I'm going to say the wrong thing, but I don't know how to say it right, but I have this magnolia in my head. But I know that's the wrong thing. But it's in my head."

I left him to rest. I couldn't listen to it yet. This brilliant man. This man who quietly spread his humble wisdom with the most gracious words. Now he couldn't distinguish between "tumor" and "magnolia."

The day went on. The next thing I remember is being in Katherine's old room. Sitting on the bed in between my mom and Peggy. My mom was telling me that there were tumors in my dad's spleen, liver, lungs, and pretty much every other internal organ. And in his brain. Then she actually said the worst. Tearfully, she looked at me and said, "The doctors think he has around six weeks to live."

My chest tightened again. Brave face gone. Sobs pouring out. They actually put a deadline on it! It's over that fast? We can't fix it? Why six weeks? Why not two years? All these questions circling around in my head and the one that actually made it out of my mouth was one of the most selfish things I could have ever said, "Who will give me away at MY wedding?"

I don't know where that came from. I didn't even have a boyfriend and had no interest in getting married any time soon. But that's the question I asked. Was I jealous of Peggy and Jane for having Dad walk them down the aisle at their weddings? Or was I jealous of all my friends in the future who would walk down the aisle with their fathers? To this day I don't know where this thought came from.

My mom threw her arms around me and held me tightly. Crying softly, she just said, "I will. I will give you away."

Then she, Peggy, and I hugged on the side of the bed until we could stop crying and go face the rest of the family.

Later, I found out just how brutal the prognosis was. The tests had been sent to an oncologist, who then forwarded the results to my parents' family physician. It was this man who broke the news. Katherine was in the room and heard the whole thing. She said it was one of the meanest ways she could imagine a doctor talking to a patient, especially one he had been treating for years. When asked about the prognosis by my parents, he simply replied, "Put it this way, at this point you need a lawyer a whole lot more than you need a doctor!"

Really?! Who says that?! He offered no hope. Chemotherapy wouldn't stop the brain tumor from growing and surgery would be impossible given the number of tumors spread throughout his body. It was time to put his affairs in order and just wait. For what? Just wait to die.

For the first time in his life, my dad took to his bed. He did not come down to the kitchen to eat his big breakfast. He did not tell stories at the dinner table. He did not go to work! Lawyers came in with wills and powers of attorney drafted, which were signed, notarized, and witnessed in the bedroom. My mom took on the business of notifying clients and arranging for them to pick up their files as the office was closing. As for me, I just wanted to go back in time to that conversation before my birthday and not warn my dad that "nobody ever said on their deathbed, 'I wish I spent more time at the office.'" Looking back, it just felt cruel that I had said that to him and I wanted nothing more than to take it back.

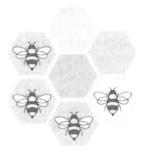

21

SOON AFTER THE DAY we got the news, we tried our best to act normal, like it wasn't the end of the world. Peggy returned to Dallas to take care of her family. Katherine went back to Virginia, where camp had already started, so it was her busy season. I let Molly and her aunt know that I would not be returning to Dallas or the mortgage company. I was going to live in Baton Rouge and take care of my parents. I had been accepted to LSU law school for the fall and was planning to stay home.

One morning, my mom approached me to run an errand for her. It seems the radiologist needed someone to pick up the MRI of my dad's brain and take it to a neurosurgeon for further evaluation. Once I was in the car with the envelope, I couldn't help but open it and look. I have never been able to understand any X-ray, MRI, ultrasound, or other images from inside the human body. However, even I was able to recognize the grapefruit sized ball in my father's head that did not belong there. I thought, "No wonder he thinks the ABCs are on the roof of his mouth and a magnolia is in his head. No one can possibly think straight with something like that in their brain." I couldn't hold back the tears as I drove the envelope to its destination and delivered it.

A few days later, I was alone in the house with my dad when the doctor called. It was the family doctor, the one with no bedside manner. He asked for my mom, but when I told him that she was not there, he asked me to put my father on the phone but for me to stay on the line and listen to the conversation so I could then repeat it to my mom.

"Red," he began, "a bright, young neurosurgeon has been reviewing your file and he would like to propose a different approach to your treatment. He swears he can surgically remove the tumor from your brain, leaving you with most of your brain intact and thinking clearly. He thinks that if the oncologists agree to follow this surgery with some aggressive chemotherapy for the tumors in your body, you can live longer than the original prognosis with a better quality of life. Now, Virginia is going to relay this conversation to Mildred and then you all let me know if you would like to meet with him further."

As soon as my mom returned home, I told her about the conversation. For the first time in weeks, my dad was downstairs at the table. He told her that he could no longer stand to just lie there in bed waiting to die and that, if there was something else for him to try, he wanted to try it. She agreed and they were off to meet the bright, young neurosurgeon.

I believe the decision to have the surgery was made when they first laid eyes on the young man. They loved his positive attitude and confidence. It was refreshing to hear such a different perspective on the treatment of this disease. But what I truly believe sold them on the surgery, when they first saw him, was his full head of thick, red hair!

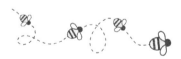

Before my dad could have the surgery to remove the brain tumor, he had to pass a physical test to see if his body could handle the procedure. I've mentioned that my father ate well and exercised. What I didn't know yet was the extent of it. Later, I found notebooks logging each day's physical activity. Whether it was "walked 4 miles," "exercise bike 45 minutes," "yard 6 hours," or even "split firewood 8 hours," all exercise was meticulously documented for years. In addition to exercise, when I was in the ninth grade, he gave up almost all sugar and fried food. My mother had to modify recipes for his desserts to be made with Equal instead of sugar. He used artificial sweetener in his iced tea. And he never added sugar to his coffee or corn flakes again.

The results of his physical had come back and the neurosurgeon announced surprisedly, "This 74-year-old man has the heart of a 28-year-old!"

Imagine that! His heart performed almost as if it was as young as mine. I wondered how this disease could spread to so many organs and begin killing him from the inside out if he was so healthy.

When it became time for the surgery, we all realized what would have to happen in the pre-op room and wondered how it would affect my dad mentally and emotionally once he left the hospital. He had always been so proud of his hair. Just a year ago, at his college 50th class reunion, he was the only man there with a full head of hair and no gray hair. The red had browned a bit over the years; however, it was still thick and full. In order to remove the brain tumor, his head would need to be shaved.

My dad made it through the brain surgery with flying colors. All of the cancerous cells had been removed from his brain. No more magnolia in his head. I was optimistic. I was ready for him to return home from the hospital with a spark in his attitude and a determination to get through chemo and conquer this disease once and for all. I was to be sadly disappointed.

After the surgery, he took to the bed again. He laid there, all day and all night. It was hard to look at his bald head with its lengthy red scar held together with metal staples through his scalp. He stopped wanting food. He never said much after that. It was as if the old Red Evans personality was left on the hospital floor in the pile of his red hair.

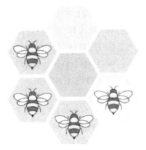

22

DURING THAT SUMMER, I tried to establish a routine in order to keep my mind off of the sickness filling our house. I mapped out a four-mile route around the neighborhood and tried to run it every day. I spent time with my law school roommate, Amie, looking for a place to rent. I had come home to Baton Rouge, but I wasn't planning to live full-time in my parents' house again. I traveled to Dallas and brought the rest of my things home. And otherwise I spent precious time with my family.

My mother, Jane, and I took on different duties in tending to my father's needs and supporting him. My mom was the only one allowed to bathe him, which she did daily. Somehow, I became the only one he would allow to shave his face. I would prop him up in the bed and sit by his side. With a warm bowl of water and a towel, I would wipe his face clean and apply the shaving cream. Then, using his vintage, double-edged, butterfly razor, I would scrape the sides of his face as gently as I could. Careful not to cut him, I would make my face into the shape I needed his to be in. "Tighten your upper lip over your top teeth like this," I would say as I delicately removed the beginnings of a mustache. Then, "Spread your lower lip and open your mouth like this," trying to get him to flatten his chin so I could go over his beard with the least amount of curves. Then, finally, I would move the razor steadily up the soft skin of his neck. When we were finished, I wiped his face again with the warm, wet towel followed by drying it with a fluffy clean one.

This shaving became our ritual and I will always treasure these moments. It's curious how such a simple act, with little to no conversation involved, can bring two people so close together. Afterwards, sometimes I would just curl up in the bed and lie next to him, silently holding his hand.

Neither of my parents was ever a big fan of taking medicine, and it became evident that this trait had not changed in my father even with the severity of his illness. He was prescribed several medications. I'm not sure what they were all supposed to treat, but I hope most were to alleviate his pain. Soon we began finding his pills stuffed between his mattress and box springs. Leaving his medicine along with a glass of water next to his bedside was no longer an option.

It was Jane who then took up medicine duty. She crushed the pills daily and mixed them into ice cream. Even though my dad had been eating less sugar for years, he always had a weakness for ice cream. His favorites were buttered pecan and homemade vanilla, but he loved them all. And though he was refusing food more often with his illness, he still managed to eat and hold down some ice cream. Jane would sit by him on the bed and gently spoon-feed him the drug-laced treat. He finished it little by little, seemingly not detecting the medicine at all.

And so together we made sure my dad was clean, shaved, and medicated. We all tried to make him eat. My mom would prepare his favorite foods, which he would turn away, uninterested. I tried to make him drink Ensure so he would at least take some nutrients into his body. Even presented chilled in a pretty glass, he rarely if ever finished one serving. He was wasting away and obviously sad and hurt. Even so, I know he had a strong faith in God and was not afraid of death. I believe he was just concerned for all of us and the pain we were going to face.

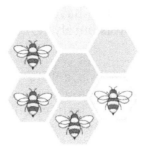

23

BILL HAD BEGUN DATING a new lady friend and they had become engaged. Upon hearing of the terminal nature of my dad's disease, he decided that the wedding date must be moved up in order for my father to attend the services. Bill insisted on being married on the 4th of July. When asked why, he replied, "That way there will always be fireworks on my anniversary." There was only one church that could accommodate this patriotic yet selfish wedding date on such late notice. It was located about twenty minutes from our home and, wait for it, the wedding would have to be at 7 a.m.

While Bill accepted the time and place restrictions on his wedding plans, he still wanted a full restaurant dinner for a reception. Not breakfast. Not brunch. He did settle on lunchtime and scheduled a full wedding dinner at a local steakhouse for noon on July 4th. This meant we were supposed to all, including my dad, be up and ready for a dawn wedding and then remain dressed up at home until it was time to go to the restaurant at noon.

The night before the wedding, Bill knocked on my bedroom door and entered. "Since it's my wedding tomorrow, I wanted to be the one to shave dad for this special occasion, if that's okay with you."

"Of course you can, have at it," I replied. I was somewhat surprised that Bill wanted to have this bonding moment with my father, but I think it was purely ceremonious, without much meaning.

The next morning, while I was getting myself ready, my mom entered my room. "Virginia, you've got to come and help your daddy! Bill is trying to shave him and he will not let him even get close! He keeps telling Bill to go away and that you are the only one who can shave his face." Of course I dropped what I was doing and tended to my father. What Bill failed to understand was that you cannot just step in and be close to someone when it's convenient for you. It took time for us to build up this shaving ritual and changing it was not something my dad was willing to allow. I shaved my dad's face, my mother dressed him in a suit—which by now was falling off of him due to his refusal to eat—and we headed to the church for the wedding.

After the service, we were all slumped over on the couches in the living room. Jane and I knew we all needed to stay dressed and ready to go back out for the noon reception, but my father was having none of that. He immediately changed and was back in the comfort of his bed while we napped for a few hours in our nice wedding clothes.

My father did not understand when my mother began dressing him up in his suit for the second time in one day, but he went along with it and we all proceeded to the restaurant. In a private room, I sat around a large table with my parents, Jane and her family, Bill, his new bride, and his new stepsons. The atmosphere was awkward as we tried to make conversation with our new in-laws, while our minds kept wandering back to my father. He looked so miserable in his baggy suit, staples still embedded in his bald head. Jane had finally had all she could take. She looked my dad in the eye and asked, "Are you ready to leave?"

Relieved, my dad simply sighed, "Yes."

Then Jane and I walked my dad to the car. I turned on the ignition and started the air conditioner, which took a while to cool off the car at noon in south Louisiana. We helped my father into the back seat of the large Chrysler sedan my mom drove at the time so he could lie down. Then we sat together in the front seats, feeling the cool air hit our faces.

"Is that better?" Jane asked him.

"Yes, it sure is. Thank you."

"We'll be home soon."

"Good."

We waited in the cool car while my mother politely finished the meal with the new in-laws before joining us for the ride home.

Later, with Dad comfortably resting back in his bed, Jane and I were quick to call the other Bees to report on how miserable our day was. We let them know that we had to go through a particular kind of torture which they had escaped simply by living elsewhere. They laughed at our recollection of the day and gave their condolences for what we had been through. Once again, Bill's behavior had tightened the bond of the Four Bees.

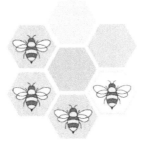

24

LATER THAT SUMMER, I returned to the house from running errands to find a fire truck and an ambulance in front of my house. I immediately got that hot, tight feeling in my chest and my pulse started racing. What had happened? Was he gone? The six weeks weren't up. He hadn't started the chemo yet. He could still get better, right?

I ran upstairs to my parents' bedroom. It seems my dad had slipped in the bathtub and, this time, he was not helping himself up at all. My mother could not lift him and carry him to bed by herself. She had him covered with towels for privacy and waited for the emergency workers to arrive with a gurney on which to carry him. He was brought away to the hospital in an ambulance.

Visiting him at the hospital was a shock to all my senses. August in Baton Rouge is hot and humid. Not just a little hot. You can shower, apply makeup, fix your hair, and dress, but as soon as you walk outside it all comes undone. The air feels like a hot, wet, towel is being wrapped around your entire body. In contrast, my dad's hospital room felt like it was thirty degrees. I found myself carrying a bag with sweatpants, sweaters, and coats with me to his room just to keep warm. Then I had to shed these layers of clothes before I reached the parking lot to be hit once again by the hot wet blanket. I just knew I was going to get pneumonia in that place.

Also, the hospital was so frigid, hard, and sterile. I had visited hospitals before, but this was different. Maternity wards are happy, children's hospitals are brightly decorated, and even surgery waiting rooms are bustling with activity. But my dad's room was in the oncology ward. People came here to die. It seemed dark. The halls were quiet and it sounded like everyone spoke in low whispers. Nurses and doctors moved delicately in and out of the rooms, checking charts and vital signs, replacing IV bags, and otherwise treating their dying patients. Although the place made me feel cold, empty, and sad, I spent as much time there with him as I could.

While in the hospital, my dad slipped in and out of consciousness. He was hooked up to machines and IV bags, as well as some sort of pump which sucked blood out of his lungs as he tried to breathe. We took turns sitting with him and occasionally speaking with him during his rare lucid moments.

I will never forget being alone with him during one of these occasions. He was awake and clear-headed when he looked directly at me and said, "No matter what happens, if you EVER decide you do not want to be a lawyer, then you do not have to be one. Always remember that." And remember, I did.

One of the oncology nurses was named Penny and she became particularly fond of my dad and our family. When she was on shift, it seemed we got extra attention and she even spent her breaks in his room getting to know our family. By this time, Katherine and Peggy had been notified of the worsening of my dad's condition and traveled to Baton Rouge to spend this time with him. Nurse Penny became particularly interested in Katherine's position at camp and the fact that they hired a camp nurse every summer. She showed interest in applying for that position in the future. I remember thinking that, if I was a nurse, I would not last long on the oncology floor and a break at a summer camp would be exactly what I would want.

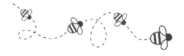

We could tell by the increasing amount of time Penny was spending in our room, even when she wasn't on her shift, that my father did not have much time left. While mom and the Four Bees surrounded him during his last days, Bill left to go on his honeymoon. Once again, my jaw just dropped at his sheer lack of empathy for anyone other than himself. Although, by this time I guess I shouldn't have been surprised. I don't even remember where they went—I think it was mountains—but I couldn't tell you if it was Colorado or Virginia. All I know is that, while the rest of the family was coming to Baton Rouge to see my dad and support my mom, Bill was on his way out of town on vacation.

We spent as much time as possible in the hospital room. Taking turns to return home to shower and change, run some errands, or grab a quick meal, we made sure someone was always there with my mom in those last days. Then, without intending to, we were all gone at the same time. I was helping Amie move a mattress into the house we were renting for law school. I believe Jane was having some small birthday party for Elizabeth. Even though she wasn't in a celebratory mood, her daughter still deserved a birthday. I'm not sure where Peggy and Katherine had gone. Anyway, there were a few hours on August 7, 1993 when my mother was alone in the room with my father. I don't know if he opened his eyes or if they had any parting words, but they had some private time together before he died peacefully with the love of his life by his side. I'm not a superstitious type, but something in me thinks he waited for us all to leave, hanging on with all the breath he could muster, just to have this time alone with Mildred Wallace Evans before he let her go and became our angel.

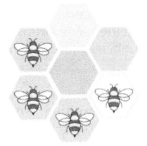

25

I HAD NEVER HAD experience with funeral planning. I'm sure not too many 24-year-olds have (excluding maybe those in the military). I was with my mother and the other Bees as she chose his casket and flowers, and wrote an obituary. He would be buried next to my brother, Jack, where they had already purchased three more burial plots. My mom wanted it over as soon as possible; therefore, visitation was scheduled for the morning of August 9th at the funeral home, with a funeral at our church that afternoon, followed by a graveside service.

The plans were set and relatives were flooding in from all over the country. The house was a flurry of activity as friends delivered vast amounts of food. Every casserole and dessert you could imagine was crammed into the two refrigerators in the house (the old one was kept down in the laundry room). Now all someone had to do was find Bill. I'm not sure who was in charge of that, but it wasn't me. I just know it was difficult to reach him on his vacation (remember, no cell phones) and he had a hard time booking a flight back to Baton Rouge in time.

Several thoughts stand out to me as I remember the day of my father's funeral. First, that it was held on what was to be my first day of law school. Amie was luckily in the same section as me and informed all the professors of the reason for my absence. The other significant detail is that my mother's next door neighbor and one of her best friends, Dot Debosier, who had spent the entire summer supporting my mom through this ordeal, lost her husband when he died suddenly on the morning of my dad's funeral. This coincidence is almost impossible to believe; however, it proved beneficial to both women as they navigated life as widows.

I also noticed that my dad seemed to have an endless number of friends. The people just kept coming. We stood in a row, hugging and shaking hands, greeting the long line of visitors at both the funeral home and the church. One man in particular stands out in my memory. He came up to me and introduced himself as a friend of my parents from the neighborhood. He told me that he often greeted my dad when he was out walking or while he was working in the yard. One afternoon, as my dad was finishing up the mowing and trimming the grass as well as sweeping or blowing off the long driveway, this man stopped to talk to him.

"It looks like you sure have been working hard today!" the man stated.

With a grin my father replied, "Well, the owner doesn't pay me very much, but sometimes she lets me sleep with her!"

I couldn't help but laugh out loud through my tears. It was such a typical Red Evans remark and I could picture the entire scene in my head.

As the visitors filed by to greet each member of the family, inevitably they would ask my mom, "I see all of your daughters, but where is Bill?" I could tell she was embarrassed, but she kept her dignity when explaining that he was flying in from out of town and expected any minute. He finally arrived after the people were seated, as the music began, and our family proceeded to take our seats in the front pews of the church.

There were hymns and prayers, but what really brought up the lump in my throat and the stinging tears in my eyes was when George Haile read a poem written by one of the architects who had spent years working for my dad in his downtown office. Through the words of the poem, I could almost feel my dad with me, smell his pipe smoke, and hear his laugh as well as his wise words of advice. I could feel his hugs and remember the feel of his hand on my forehead if he came home from work to find out that I was in bed with a fever. The words brought to life the man for whom everyone had come to mourn. I held my mother's hand and just let myself absorb the poem and all the feelings it evoked.

When the service was over and the family stood to walk down the aisle and exit the church, my mother slipped her arm through mine, almost as if I was leading her down the aisle. I think that's when I changed. As the youngest child, I was no longer the baby. I was taking care of her now. It was time for me to be the grown-up.

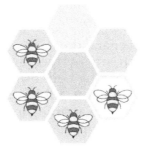

26

WHEN I LOOK BACK at the last year of my dad's life, I see that he lived freely and happily. He did more with family and traveled and genuinely enjoyed life.

Each year at Christmas, besides all my mother's decorations, one of the things I looked forward to the most was watching my mom open the gifts from my dad. These were not gifts of exquisite jewelry or furs. In fact, sometimes they were quite ordinary and mundane, such as a 6-inch skillet or a new toilet seat. But the excitement was not about the actual present. Attached to each present was a poem. Written in his perfectly spaced, block letters. Each poem rhymed and each contained some sort of riddle or hint meant to help the reader try to guess the present inside. Every year I just loved to sit on the floor at her feet and watch the joy on my mother's face as she read the poems and tried to guess the gift. Then we would all usually fall out with laughter when she opened it and we saw what it was.

For Christmas of 1992, I remember the poem was especially long. It spoke of all the adventures he and my mom had gone through during the year. It recounted moving the office from downtown to home and finishing the drawing room, remodeling some of the master bathroom, the 50th reunion of the LSU class of 1942, and of course the family vacation to Washington D.C. and Williamsburg. He had inadvertently made the last year of his life one of his best.

I think the gift that year was a sterling silver platter that my mother had been eyeing; however, it was packed in a box from a new toilet seat and then carefully wrapped. With all the joy he had given her that year, I'm sure she would have been happy with another new toilet seat. But she was certainly surprised by the platter. That year, he also gave her a gold chain with a pendant which was a coin from 1942 framed in gold. She continued to wear that reminder of the year she married Red for the rest of her life.

My dad's poems and written words are a treasure for all of us to hold on to and preserve. They bring me strength and comfort and fill my heart with his love even now.

In fact, one time when I was going through an extremely difficult time in my own marriage and life, I was wandering around my house alone, sobbing loudly, and yelling at God, "Are you even there? Can't you see what I'm going through? Can't you just show me some kind of sign that you even care about me?"

Suddenly, I felt a strange calm as my eyes drifted up to the top shelf of a dusty bookcase in my house. I reached up to the far corner of the top shelf and pulled down a book. It ended up being one of my dad's Bibles. Then a slip of paper fell out of the Bible and onto the floor. I picked it up and immediately recognized the writing—the same perfectly spaced, block lettering. It had been written on the back of a page of an old deposition (remember, he was way ahead of his time when it came to recycling). Right when I needed to feel God's presence the most, I read the words my father had written and stored in his Bible:

Full half a hundred times I've sobbed,
'I can't go on, I can't go on.'
And yet full half a hundred times
I've hushed my sobs, and gone.
My answer, if you ask me how,
May seem presumptuously odd,
But I think that what kept keeping on
When I could not, was God.

Every time one of us experienced a strange coincidence, blessing, or miracle, my father would say, "You know, I think Somebody besides people had something to do with that." I know that Somebody besides people led my eyes to the corner of that top, dusty shelf. Finding that Bible, his favorite passages underlined, notes in the margins, and the handwritten poem tucked inside, was indeed a miracle.

That day, I dropped to the floor holding the paper, both crying and thanking God for showing me this poem and for all the extraordinary love in my life. And especially for my sisters, who are always there for me no matter what circumstances life may have in store.

Later, when Jane hit a rough patch in her life, I gave her the Bible with the poem in it. Since then, we trade it back and forth whenever either of us is going through a difficult season and needs some encouragement. It's at my house now.

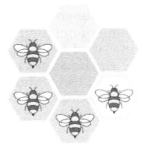

27

WHILE I HAD SPENT most of my life believing I would not be able to go on living without my parents, I was learning to cope. After my father's funeral, we all tried to move forward with our lives even though his loss left an emptiness which we all felt. My mother strung her wedding ring along with my father's onto the gold chain with the 1942 coin. I believe these emblems, dangling just above her heart, gave her comfort that he was always with her.

For me, things began to move quickly after the funeral. I started attending law school the next day. I had no idea what I was getting into. I was overwhelmed by the amount of reading which was expected of us every night, in five different subjects. Unlike college, where I treated attendance as an option and was able to cram large amounts of information at the last minute, law school was different. The professors called roll and had a seating chart. You were only allowed a limited number of absences and if you exceeded this limit, you would fail. Also, the professors used the Socratic method, meaning they called on students at random and asked questions about the assigned readings, and we were expected to answer in front of the whole class.

This type of teaching was extremely intimidating to me. While I was loud and confident among my family and friends, I was shy and uncomfortable speaking in a room full of fellow law students. This was made worse by the fact that I always felt as if I was one or two steps behind everyone else in the class. I did not really understand the meaning of the cases we were assigned to read until after they had been discussed in the class and I had taken a copious amount of notes on the subject. Thus, when called upon to answer in class, I felt knots in my stomach and a huge lump in my throat, which seemed to prevent my breathing as well as my speech. I would feebly mumble an answer, which was usually some short statement in an attempt to satisfy the professors and have them move on to someone else.

While I did not enjoy most of my classes in law school and hated the amount of homework, I still managed to have fun. It was great to be back in town with my old college friends. Amie and I had several parties and invited all of our friends from undergrad over. (That first year we did not associate with many of our law classmates.) The house we rented was across the street from a fast food burger place. While we didn't care for their food, the employees would let us come over and take rows of the little paper cups used for the ketchup dispenser. We would use the cups to make a variety of flavors of Jell-O shots for our friends to enjoy.

One great benefit to being a law student at LSU was that our student section in Tiger Stadium had much better seats than those of the undergraduates. And we were allowed to purchase two season tickets instead of one. I could now bring a friend to the games with me who was not in law school. Once again, I was able to hear the band and the roar of the fans, and smell the bourbon and Sprite, while cheering on my favorite football team.

One of the greatest things about that first year back home was that my nephew, Aaron, had decided to come to LSU that year. For the first time in our lives, we attended the same school. I remember one game when Peggy and Tim came down to visit him. We all had a big tailgate party before the LSU game. There was a miniature keg of beer called a "party ball" and plenty of alcohol and mixers for other drinks. And, of course, we had tons of food. Jane even made sure we had purple and gold iced petit fours from one of the best bakeries for dessert. LSU ended up losing that game to Florida by a score of 58-3, but because our family was together, we still enjoyed every minute of it.

Sometimes I would pick up Aaron from his dorm on Sunday and take him to my mom's house for a visit. He would bring loads of laundry, which she would wash and dry, while we ate home-cooked meals like turkey or roast with rice and gravy and all the sides. I believe she enjoyed cooking and taking care of others like she had taken care of my dad for the last fifty years. By late Sunday we would leave with full bellies, clean clothes, and a little extra spending money, which she would slip to us as we said goodbye.

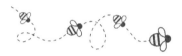

My immediate dive into law school kept me so busy that it served as a distraction from the recent loss of my father. My mother also needed to find distractions in order to stay active and busy. She was not one to sit around all day and cry or mourn her loss.

One day she looked outside to see Bill pulling up the driveway in a U-Haul truck. He had been living in Virginia for over a year, so she wondered what on earth he was moving that needed so much space. Imagine her surprise when he came in and starting picking and choosing things from her house to take back with him. When he started taking down my dad's drawing table, she exclaimed, "And just where do you think you are going with that?"

"Well, Dad isn't here. And you don't need it. And I wanted something of his." He had also taken down a limited edition framed baseball poster which had been presented to my father during a game at Alex Box stadium, since his friend and roommate did not have descendants of his own to accept it.

"Put that picture down and don't touch that drawing table! You're not taking anything. In case you haven't noticed, I'M not dead yet!"

"Well, I just thought I could have it. You don't need all this stuff."

"I said put it down and get out. And don't ever take anything out of this house!"

And that was that. He went back to Virginia without a U-Haul full of my dad's things.

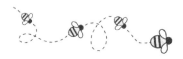

While she no longer prepared the enormous breakfast or full course dinners for my father every day, she took her food preparation talents to a much larger level. She became in charge of Wednesday Night Supper at our church. She took this job seriously. She spent her time planning the menu, shopping for the ingredients—some wholesale bulk amounts and some retail. She would begin preparing the food by at least Tuesday, and by Wednesday night everyone from the congregation would file in line in the fellowship hall at the church to buy one of Mildred Evans' dinner plates. Amie and I would go to these church suppers as often as we could, as it was much better than anything we would cook up from our freezer or get from a fast food joint.

Church volunteering was certainly not her only activity and she was to remain busy even without my father's office work to attend to. She volunteered as a docent at the newly-built LSU Lod Cook Alumni Center and was later asked to serve on the board of the LSU Retired Teachers Association. She had a weekly bridge game with several of her friends and continued her clubs like PEO, among others. And, as always, she went to the beauty parlor every Thursday morning to have her hair done and take in the latest gossip.

After her neighbor Dot Debosier's husband died on the morning of my dad's funeral, they began to travel together. They would drive down to LaRose, Louisiana on the Bayou to visit my Uncle Charlie, who would spend the afternoon feeding them his home-cooked Cajun fare and entertain them with stories that could keep anyone laughing for hours. Without my father by her side, she would bring Dot with her to attend the reunions of his army company, the 529th. I believe Dot met more friends and enjoyed these reunions as much as my mother did.

Without my father around, she also loosened up a bit. Not that they were ever big teetotalers, but my parents weren't exactly party animals. I only remember drinking with my father once. It was at a wedding reception in which Jane had been a bridesmaid. As my mother worked the room chitchatting with everyone she knew, my dad and I stood by the bar in the corner. He eventually ordered straight Jack Daniels and I ordered one with Sprite in it. We ended up standing in that corner most of the night and had more than one refill. I remember in these situations he would always say, "If we could just find your mother a job where she could get paid by the word, we'd be millionaires!" It was hard to peel her away from any social situation where she had friends to talk to.

After his death, she began traveling with Dot Debosier to the Mississippi Gulf Coast casinos. While my dad drank alcohol on occasion, he never gambled. I remember if anyone bought a lottery ticket he would proudly announce, "I still have my dollar!" Now, my mom was free to play. She loved the slot machines and would eagerly ride the tour bus with rolls of nickels tucked into her purse in anticipation of hitting the winning jackpot. Jane and I would always laugh when she would talk about her adventures at the "*casina.*" She pronounced it as if it ended with an "a" instead of an "o." (She also started to branch out from her regular coffee to enjoy a "*cappucina.*") Dot would arrange many group casino trips for the elderly and always brought my mom along as a roommate and willing participant.

My mother also began traveling with her former college roommate, Dot Howell. These trips did not center around gambling, but consisted of marvelous sightseeing adventures. They traveled to New England in the fall when the leaves were changing and bursting with color. (Baton Rouge only has two seasons—summer and winter, with no beauty to observe in the transition). They took an Alaskan cruise in the summer where she was able to see the whales, mountains, and extraordinary scenery from both the ship and a glass-encased train with full views of the surrounding landscape. They also made a few trips to Branson, Missouri to soak up the entertainment and energy.

Mom started going out to Mexican restaurants with us. I don't know if my dad just didn't care for Mexican food, but we did not grow up eating tacos or dining out at Mexican restaurants. Now it was something she loved to do and she always ordered a frozen margarita as soon as the waitress approached the table. I don't remember her drinking alcohol before my father died, but afterwards she enjoyed her share of frozen margaritas whenever the opportunity arose.

During this time of traveling and activities, I remember that whenever anyone would ask her what she was going to do now that she wasn't working at my dad's office, my mother would straighten up her back and grin, saying, "Why, I'm going to spend my children's inheritance!"

While she stayed busy with activities, clubs, and travel, my mom always had time for family. The holidays did not change after the loss of my father. In fact, that first Christmas after his death, she went all-out on her decorations and parties as usual. Without my dad to direct the setting up of the giant Christmas tree, we had to have family and several neighbors over to help with the process. It was right after Thanksgiving and one of those hot muggy days that still show up in Baton Rouge no matter what month it is. As we stood outside holding the tree up with ropes to make sure it was straight while another neighbor nailed the stand to the trunk of the tree, everyone was swatting at mosquitoes, which seemed to be eating us alive.

Once the stand was on the tree, it was time to drag it into the house and hoist it upright. Jane and I held the ropes tied to the top of the tree from the balcony and pulled while everyone at the bottom pushed up the base of the tree until it was standing. Hot, mosquito-bitten, and dripping with sweat, we all admired the tall Frasier fir before we noticed that Bill had stayed inside the entire time. Without lifting a finger to help, he was lounged back in the blue La-Z-Boy recliner with a giant bowl of ice cream. If I hadn't witnessed it with my own eyes, I never would have believed someone could be that lazy, not making a move to help his mother while friends and neighbors readily labored for her. But he was always ready and able to eat any food she had prepared.

Mom decorated the large tree in the family room as well as the smaller one in the living room with its vast collection of snow village houses arranged beneath it. She still hosted the Sunday school class Christmas party. She continued to shop for everyone and make sure Santa came to fill our stockings and supply numerous gifts under the tree. I could hear her gulping down a sob and see her blink away tears as she pulled out the stockings which read "Jack" and "Red" before gently placing them back in the storage box. Our group was getting smaller and there would be two less stockings, fewer gifts, and no beautifully printed poems on packages for her to open this year.

28

AFTER HIS FRESHMAN YEAR, Aaron returned to Dallas to attend University of North Texas. I don't blame him. LSU is a huge school and, for someone not from Baton Rouge with a set of high school friends and home nearby, it's easy to get swallowed up. And maybe he's a little like me.

After my first year of law school, my mother decided the house was too big for her to stay in alone; however, she did not want to move out. So my father's brilliant design for the addition to the new house turned out to be useful. It was decided that my mother would live in the new part. The old house would be separated from the new addition, the closets and hallway between them would be demolished, and a new kitchen would be added to the old house. Soon work was being done and Jane and her family moved into the newly remodeled "old house" next door to my mother. I think it was a good arrangement. Jane was able to live in the neighborhood of her childhood and my mother would have family on one side and a best friend on the other side. She would not be completely alone.

At the beginning of the summer of 1994, before camp started, Katherine and I made another trip to Hilton Head, South Carolina. However, this time, instead of flying, I drove my

Jeep Wrangler the entire 12 hours across Mississippi, Alabama, Florida, and part of Georgia to get there. We stayed in the same place with the screen porch overlooking the beach. It was nice to just relax in the sun and enjoy the ocean after a year of reading and studying. On the last night of the trip, all the doors and windows were stolen off of my Jeep. I was devastated. I had parked that car uncovered behind a rental house in a high-crime area of Baton Rouge for a year with no incident. Then I take it to an exclusive resort island and this happens. I made the long drive home with the cold wind freezing my body and the heater on full blast seeming only to burn my feet. It was one of the longest and hardest road trips of my life.

When I got home, my mother accompanied me to the Chrysler dealership she had dealt with for most of fifty years. Chrysler now sold Jeeps, so we were there to find out the cost of new doors and windows for the Wrangler and get them ordered. Now was her chance to get back at my dad for saying yes to that car. While the manager was supposedly looking up the replacement cost for my Wrangler's missing parts, his coworker started showing us Jeep Cherokees. My mom thought these small SUVs were much safer than the open-air Wranglers. And she must have prepared him, because he even remarked that if I were to trade in my Wrangler for one of these, my monthly payment would remain the same amount. Before I knew what had happened, I was driving home in a gold Jeep Cherokee, never to see my precious Jeep Wrangler again except in the pictures my dad took from the ladder that day in the driveway.

My next two years of law school were not much different from my first year. I was busy with classes and homework, spending time with college friends, and visiting my mom as often as possible. In September of my third year of law school, ten years after Jane's daughter, Elizabeth, was born, Jane had a baby boy. She named him Jack Watson, after our brother, and after my dad's grandmother, Virginia Caroline Watson. It was a joy to have a new life in the family and I believe my mother took to him more than she had the older grandchildren. I don't believe she loved him any more than the others. But having him next door provided her the opportunity to spend more time with him. I also think she loved that there was a precious new "Jack" in her life. She spent time reading to him in the blue La-Z-Boy or, as he got older, went to Jane's house and sat with him as he played Nintendo video games.

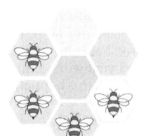

29

ALTHOUGH I DIDN'T PARTICULARLY care for the homework or the content, I enjoyed the life of being a law student much more than that of working at the mortgage company. As the third year came to an end, I was once again forced to think about my future. I needed to study for and pass the bar exam and then begin looking for a job as an attorney. But I wasn't ready to be grown-up yet. Why couldn't things just stay the way they were? Why couldn't I have my dad and brother back and live in my old room and be taken care of by my parents?

Why was transition and growing so hard for me? I was afraid: afraid of failing, of not being good enough, of not becoming someone Red and Mildred Evans would be proud of.

My law school graduation in May of 1996 was scheduled to be the morning before Charlotte would graduate from high school in Dallas. My mother came to watch my ceremony, which I considered mediocre at best. The dean of the law school spent his entire time on the stage praising the top ten percent of the class and how much he enjoyed his breakfasts and lunches with them and how he appreciated the time he spent getting to know them. In the meantime, the man had never met me or most of the other ninety percent of the graduates he failed to mention.

I was ready for it to be over and to get away from the place by then.

After my graduation ceremony, my mother and I changed clothes and I drove her in her car to Dallas to attend Charlotte's graduation. We arrived at Peggy's house in the early evening, excited to see everyone and celebrate another milestone for one of my nieces. My mom stayed at Peggy's house while I had Molly pick me up so I could sleep at her house. She was still working at the mortgage company, but had earned several promotions since I had left and was now an executive. I spent the night catching up with her and headed back up to Peggy's house in Allen the next evening.

It's true that everything is bigger in Texas, and that applies to high school graduations. Charlotte's class must have been ten times larger than my high school class. The ceremony was in a huge gymnasium with graduates seated in chairs on the floor and families in the stands. It took a long time to read off all the names and watch as they went on stage to accept their diplomas. But she was graduating with honors and was heading to the University of Texas, and we were all so proud to be there.

After the ceremony, we returned to Peggy's house to celebrate. Tim popped open a bottle of champagne and poured glasses for everyone as he proposed a toast.

"Charlotte, put that glass down!" Peggy exclaimed. "Tim, she's not even 21. She can't have that."

"Aw, come on Peg, it's just a tiny bit and it's her graduation."

"No. She is not old enough to drink and she cannot have that."

And so we all, except Charlotte and Peggy, raised our glasses and toasted Charlotte's achievement. It felt so awkward, but the matter was settled and there was no use arguing about it.

Molly picked me up soon afterwards and we headed back to her house. Charlotte and a friend had plans to go out with Aaron and one of his friends. She had been telling him that all she wanted from him for graduation was a night on the town with her big brother. However, somehow he lost her and she ended up with no place to go. Frustrated with Aaron, she called me and I invited her over to Molly's house.

Charlotte and her friend ended up spending their graduation night with a couple of 27-year-olds on a deck on the back of Molly's house in Plano, Texas. But the night ended up being one of my most fun memories with her. Before that night, I had been in social situations with Aaron, but only in family situations with Charlotte. We stayed up half of the night discussing books, art, theater, and surprisingly, sports. I remember that, as a drama major and supporter of the arts, Charlotte did not see much value in athletics. Molly, who had played tennis throughout high school and college, discussed the self-discipline, teamwork, time management, and hard work ethic that she was able to bring from her tennis experience into her life and career. From that night on, whether we were in Baton Rouge, Dallas, or later New York, I always valued my conversations with Charlotte as thought-stimulating and fair-minded as well as downright funny. She was now initiated as an official BIT (Bitch-In-Training) and I decided that someday she was going to be a full Bee like my sisters and me.

The next morning, as we prepared to leave Peggy's house, we noticed that my mom's lower leg and foot were swollen to more than twice their normal size. She was in obvious pain and needed medical attention. However, she wanted to go home to Baton Rouge rather than see a new doctor in Texas. I situated her in the back seat of the car, lying down, with the swollen leg propped up on the back of her seat. I must have driven that car over 90 miles per hour all the way from Dallas to Baton Rouge, trying not to panic but determined to get her to a doctor in time.

I'm not sure if we called her regular doctor or if I took her straight to the hospital. All I know is that she was hospitalized once again for blood clots. After five years with no breast cancer, her doctor had taken her off of tamoxifen. Since tamoxifen was determined to be the cause of her previous blood clots, it made sense to them to have her stop taking her blood thinner, Coumadin, at the same time. This turned out to be a bad mistake. Now her leg was filled with blood clots, swollen and painful.

She spent another two weeks in the hospital on IV blood thinners under the supervision of doctors until the clots broke up. Then, as a safety measure, the doctors performed a surgery on her during which they inserted a filter in the vein leading up from her legs to her heart and lungs. This filter would serve to prevent any future clots which might form in her legs from traveling up into any vital organs of her body, such as her heart, lungs, or brain. While it was simply a preventive procedure, it was still surgery, and we were all worried. Here I was with my mother, at the hospital, being the one to listen to the doctors and try to understand her plan of care. I was learning more and more that things were going to change and I was going to be the grown-up now.

She continued to take Coumadin for most of the remainder of her life. This required frequent trips to the doctor for bloodwork to adjust the dosage. She needed to be much more careful, especially when traveling. She was told to stop every hour and walk around rather than stay seated for hours at a time. Not an easy adjustment when your favorite activities are bus rides to the casino, road trips all over the country, playing bridge, and sitting with your baby grandson. But she was always positive and accepted her circumstances with a smile and refused to complain. That was Mildred. She did not want to be sick because she did not want any pity or attention to be on her. She wanted to be independent and take care of herself as well as continue to take care of everyone else.

30

THAT SUMMER, AFTER MY mother returned home from the hospital, I spent my time studying for the bar exam. For the first time in my life, I seriously studied. I was determined to pass this exam on the first try. I told myself I was only going to go through this once and, if I failed, I was not meant to be a lawyer and I would try to get a job as a flight attendant—never mind that I got anxiety every time I got on an airplane. I had just heard that flight attendants earn a good salary with great benefits, including free flights. I threw myself into studying full-time, but had my backup plan ready.

The Louisiana bar exam consists of nine separate tests on different areas of the law. Each test was a two- -and-a-half-hour essay exam. The tests were administered as three essay exams given on Monday, Wednesday, and Friday in the last week of July. Tuesday and Thursday were days to rest and cram for the following day's three tests. All the information learned over three years of school would be covered on the exam, and therefore had to be condensed and memorized prior to that week.

Amie and I had a strict schedule which we stuck to for the whole summer. I would wake up at 7 each morning and study a particular subject until noon. This consisted of condensing all my notes on that particular area of law into an outline. At noon, Amie would arrive at my house and we would spend the afternoon working through old exams on that day's topic. We would then discuss our answers to the test, take notes on what was right or wrong about our answers, then work another old exam. We would continue to do this until at least 6 p.m. At 7:30 p.m. I would run at least three miles. Despite the summer heat, this was necessary for me to release my pent-up stress and try to tire out my body after drinking coffee all day to get through the studying.

We repeated this exact routine every day throughout the summer of 1996. Each day we moved to a different topic. Once we had been through all nine, we started over again, condensing outlines to smaller bullets of information each time and trying to commit everything to memory. In all of my years as a student, I don't believe I was ever as disciplined or put as much effort into preparing for anything.

When the week of the exam arrived, we met in the parking lot and crammed each outline into our brains one last time. By then each subject had been condensed into a one page outline, front and back. We'd go inside the arena downtown where the exam was administered, take the test, then head to the parking lot for a quick snack while we crammed for the next essay test. The week was mentally and physically exhausting and we made plans to go out and celebrate big after the last day. By the time we finished on Friday, we headed over to the Pastime Lounge downtown to start drinking. I believe we each managed to keep our eyes open for one beer before we admitted to ourselves that all we wanted to do was go home and sleep for a week.

Although I didn't have a huge night out after finishing the bar exam, I felt relieved and satisfied when it was over. I knew for the first time that I had done absolutely everything I could do to prepare for that test and, if I didn't pass, then I just wasn't meant to be a lawyer. I would go ahead and start my new job as a law clerk and wait for the results, which would not be released until October.

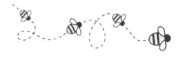

In the fall of 1996, I began clerking for a district judge. The job did not pay much and the district covered three parishes, requiring me to drive to Livingston, Amite, and Greensburg, Louisiana on a regular basis. I was basically on my own; however, with the meager salary, rent, and now student loans to repay, my cash flow was low. For that year, my mom continued to let me use her Exxon card to buy gas, which was necessary with the amount of driving my new job entailed. I remember during that year the gas price went above $1.00 per gallon and I was appalled!

The first thing I learned as a judicial law clerk was that law school had taught me nothing about how to be a lawyer. Watching what really happened in the courtroom, from civil motions, criminal arraignments, plea agreements, civil commitments, and trials, I realized that all of the theory I had memorized for the bar exam was completely useless in the courtroom. I saw that some of the best attorneys were not from the top ten percent of the class and that successful lawyers knew how to deal with people. They needed to communicate well with their clients and be able to convincingly make their points known to their opposing counsel and the judge. Most of all, they needed to treat the judge's staff and all court personnel with respect. If an attorney was rude or mean to any member of the staff, it was made known to the judge and it would take that lawyer a long time to rebuild any kind of positive reputation in that court in the future.

This was a great way to be introduced into the true practice of law. A test to see if it was for me. Especially because judges in this district handled both civil and criminal matters, which meant I was able to observe a variety of different types of practice. But above all, it was fun. I became close friends with the entire staff for our division and with the other law clerks. We frequently joined each other for happy hours after work or nights out in Baton Rouge. I was once again the loud and funny one, but never afraid to laugh at myself.

I remember one particular jury trial in a civil case. As one of the attorneys was presenting his closing argument to the jury, I was handed a telephone message to deliver to the judge who was presiding from the bench. Dressed in my nice skirt and blazer, I tried to discreetly sneak across the courtroom so as not to interrupt the attorney's well-rehearsed speech to the jury. Then, without knowing what was happening, I missed a step and fell down right on my butt and then my back in the middle of the courtroom. After flailing around on my back, in my skirt, I was finally able to stand and recover my balance. The members of the jury began howling with laughter while I stood red-faced and walked the message to the judge. I felt so humiliated. However, one of the jurors approached me that evening, after their verdict was read, and said, "I just want to thank you so much for that fall. I had not been able to keep my eyes open listening to that man talk, and your fall was the perfect jolt of entertainment we needed to wake up and pay attention."

"You're quite welcome," I replied. "I'm so glad I was able to help."

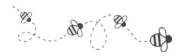

We still did not have internet or cell phones when our bar exam results were released. While letters were sent to us in the mail, the results were immediately posted on the window of the Louisiana Supreme Court building in New Orleans. I remember the judge taking me and some other clerks out for drinks the night before, then giving us the next day off in case we felt the urge to drive down to New Orleans to check them instead of waiting for the snail mail. I woke the next morning, feeling wiped out from the night before, but ready to make the drive. Just before I left, a friend of mine who was working in New Orleans called to congratulate me.

"You passed all nine parts on the first try!" she exclaimed.

"No way. How can you tell?"

"I just saw it on the Supreme Court window."

"But we had to use secret names. You didn't know mine. And I know you don't have my Social Security number."

"They only post the secret names of the people who failed or conditioned (meaning they passed some parts, but would have to retake other parts in February). They use the real names for the people who passed. Call them if you don't believe me."

"No. I believe you if you really saw it on there. I'm just in shock. I'm so excited. And I'm also glad I don't have to drive to New Orleans today."

I felt so relieved. Maybe I had a little regret that I would not get to experience the adventure of becoming a flight attendant, but that passed quickly. I still had the day off, so I was going to relax. I phoned my mom to tell her the news, then went back to bed, knowing my clerkship would be over in less than a year and I would have to start looking for a job as a real lawyer.

I spent the entire spring sending resumes to firms all over Baton Rouge and even New Orleans while continuing to clerk for the judge. One thing about Louisiana: there is no shortage of lawyers. The state has four law schools cranking out more of them every year and the job market is highly competitive. While I was interviewed by several firms, I received more rejection letters than I want to remember. It was a humiliating experience.

Towards the end of the summer, I finally received an offer from a small firm in downtown Baton Rouge. I'm not sure if they were impressed by my credentials or if I was hired because the senior partner had been best friends with my judge in law school. Regardless of how I got the job, the people seemed nice, I loved the building, and the work was going to be interesting. It was time to say goodbye to my court coworkers and begin working on the other side of the bench.

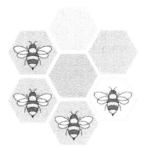

31

BETWEEN MY LAST WEEK as a law clerk and my first week as a lawyer, my life encountered two major events. First, I got engaged to be married. I was thrilled. I began buying all the bridal magazines that I never had allowed myself to buy before. I thought of the planning that needed to be done. And soon. I had always wanted a Christmas wedding. I wanted everything at my mom's house to be decorated the way it always had been. And of course, any church or reception hall would already be fully decorated for the holidays. In my mind, I pictured my mother and me going shopping for gowns, flowers, cakes, photographers, bridesmaids' dresses, and all the other activities that went into planning. My dad might not be there to give me away, but my mother and I could handle the whole thing together.

Right after my engagement, back at my mom's house, she informed me that the doctor had discovered an aneurysm on her aorta and that she would be going into the hospital for emergency surgery the next morning. She showed me where she kept a key to her safety deposit box and she informed me that she had had the locks changed to her house. She gave me new keys to give to my sisters and to her next door neighbor, and under no circumstances was Bill to get one of these keys. "This must be serious," I thought, "She's acting like she might die." I had no idea what an aortic aneurysm was, but I was about to find out.

We notified the Bees and they came swarming in. Bill and his wife also came in town. We waited anxiously in the waiting room at the hospital for the surgeon to give some news. Of course, Pastor George Haile was with us, as he had always been during any crisis.

The doctor came into the private family waiting room and began explaining the procedure and results. I listened carefully and tried to absorb everything that was happening. Bill took over as if he had been in charge of us all his life. He asked all of the questions and took all of the instructions and then started barking orders at all of us about what we needed to do.

I was beginning to realize how serious the situation was and how close my mother had come to death. And her condition was still critical. I don't know why they did not keep her in an intensive care unit; however, they moved her to a regular hospital room and we all surrounded her bedside. Bill was saying that his wife used to be a nurse and knew the most about everything and should be the one in charge. He said someone always needed to be there and continued bossing us around.

I couldn't keep my mouth shut. Filter gone. I pulled him out of her room and into the hallway. "You have not lifted a finger to help your mother since you showed up late to her husband's funeral! Then you come into town barking orders at those of us that have been with her this whole time."

He wasted no time screaming at me. I don't even remember all the words he used. I just know it was a loud fight. Too loud for a hospital. Our cousin, who had basically been raised by my parents, stepped in between us, finally separating us and calming everyone down. It was decided that someone needed to be in Mom's hospital room around the clock. My cousin drafted a chart assigning everyone shifts to stay with her, for how long we did not yet know, but she wasn't coming home soon. He made sure that Bill and I never had a shift next to one another so that we wouldn't have to cross paths. I left the hospital, knowing I would be back, but not knowing if or when I would have to see Bill again.

Unfortunately for her, Katherine was the next one to have to confront him. While Mom was in the hospital, Katherine was staying in her house. She pulled into the driveway after a long shift at the hospital to find Bill angrily standing in the front yard.

"I've been trying to get in the house for hours. Why won't my key work?" he demanded to know.

"Mom changed the locks so your key wouldn't work and we were given specific instructions not to let you in."

Wow. Now it was Katherine's turn to have the confrontation. I don't remember all the exact words as she told the story to us, but apparently, they had a screaming match in the front yard until he gave up and left in frustration. She made sure not to use her new key to open the door until he was long gone. He wouldn't be taking any of my parents' things on this trip.

My shifts in the hospital were long and quiet. I had checked in with my new law firm. They gave me a file and informed me that, on my first day of work, I was to drive to court in Jena, a small Louisiana town a couple of hours drive from Baton Rouge, for a hearing. What? I had to go to court on my first day at work? Alone? I was terrified. I took the file to the hospital and began studying everything about it while listening to my mom's quiet breathing. It ended up being a pretty easy task; however, as a baby lawyer, I was scared to actually go to court and appear on behalf of a client.

When I wasn't reading the file for my court appearance, I was looking through bridal magazines. It was August and I needed to get to work if I was going to plan a wedding for this Christmas. I thought back to Jane's wedding, to the fight she had with Bill in the bathroom as she tried to get ready. I thought of all the complaints and fights with him in Washington D.C. and Williamsburg. And I was still so irritated at him about the fight in the hall of the hospital. I realized that, every time he was near me, I felt stressed and agitated. I wanted my wedding day to be peaceful and fun. I did not want him trying to take charge or tell people what to do. I didn't want him bothering my mom, making her work for him while he didn't lift a finger to help her. I decided that it would be my special day, and that for it to turn out calm and pleasant, it would be best not to invite him. I made that decision in my mom's hospital room as her aorta was healing, and I never regretted it.

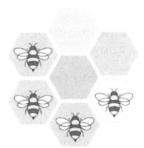

32

ONCE MY MOM GOT home from the hospital, she became excited about planning the wedding. She did not have all of her energy back and was somewhat weaker than she had been, but that was to be expected after such a major surgery. We were all just so lucky the aneurysm was caught early and that she survived the event. And I was so grateful to have her to help me plan, especially since I wanted a Christmas wedding.

Rule number one when planning a wedding in the South: CHECK THE FOOTBALL SCHEDULE! In Baton Rouge, we didn't have a great live theater like the big cities, there are no mountains or beaches for recreation, and we don't even have the Big Easy party atmosphere of New Orleans. But what we have that no other city has: seven or eight Saturdays every fall in LSU Tiger Stadium.

People spend a lot of money on tickets to these home games. Then they invest heavily in their tailgate setup. You have to have the perfect spot, a parking pass, food, drinks, and now satellite TVs showing all the other SEC games going on during the day while you wait for the kickoff on Saturday night—unless CBS picks up the game and puts it during the day, which everyone hates. Everyone looks forward to these Saturdays all year long.

You can end up being the least popular person in town if you do not schedule your personal events around LSU football.

In 1997, LSU was not expected to be playing very well or end up a highly ranked team. But, you never know what miracles can happen, so I chose a date that avoided every LSU game and also made sure the date would not conflict with the SEC Championship game. Who knows, maybe that could have been our year? And besides, everyone likes to watch the other SEC games even when LSU is not playing. Therefore, the date had to be Saturday, December 13th. Everything would be decorated for Christmas and nobody would have to miss any football to be there. Step one complete.

Since my mom had been sick, I did most of the other planning on my own. I tried on dresses in New Orleans and Baton Rouge. I never realized how expensive wedding dresses could be. I settled on one from Goudchaux's for about one fourth the price of the cheapest one I could find at the boutique wedding shops in New Orleans.

Next step, I walked naively into a local bakery and asked to order a wedding cake. I thought that's what you did. I'd ordered birthday cakes before, it can't be that hard.

"Do you have an appointment?" the woman behind the counter asked.

"Um, no. Do I need one?"

She looked at me as if I had asked her to make a cockroach pie. She was so rude and snobby about it. "Yes, you MUST have an appointment, when is your wedding?"

"December 13."

"Of this year?"

"Yes ma'am. Is that a problem?"

"I should think so! That's just impossible. We don't have any available appointments for over a month, and we are booked for wedding cakes for over six months. You should have made an appointment a year ago."

I left the bakery defeated. I wondered if this was how everything was going to work. How could I be so stupid? And why was I trying to do all of this without my mother? Weren't you supposed to have your mom with you to do all of the wedding planning? I decided not to give up yet.

Luckily, a friend of mine knew a lady who made wedding cakes out of her house, and when I called her, she was available to have a cake ready for my date. Next step, photographer. I knew a girl from high school who was a local wedding photographer, so I called her. She wasn't available, but referred me to one who was and I hired him on the spot using the little money I had been able to save as a law clerk.

I did bring my mom with me to the florist. She always had a green thumb and knew everything about plants and flowers. We walked into the small shop that she had always used. They were very sweet to us and didn't require us to make an appointment to come back. Their first question was what color were the bridesmaids' dresses. "What? I don't know. Does that matter?" I was shocked at my naivete once again. No wonder people hire wedding planners.

"I don't have any dresses picked out yet. Can you just make everything 'Christmassy'? You know, reds, greens, maybe some holly, but not prickly? And my bouquet can just be white?"

And so, with just that little bit of information, they took my flower order and agreed to deliver them on December 13. They didn't turn out as I had pictured in my mind, but I couldn't complain. After all, I didn't give them any clue about what I expected or even show them a picture from a magazine similar to what I really wanted.

I was in court in New Orleans one morning and, once the hearing was over, I stopped in Saks Fifth Avenue. In the formal dress section, I found a nice, plain, formal gown that was on sale. They had sizes left in all the sizes I would need for my local bridesmaids. They checked the Dallas and Chicago stores which had the sizes for my out-of-town bridesmaids. So I bought up the ones in New Orleans and instructed them to hold on to the others. My wedding party would be wearing long, navy blue shift gowns from Saks Fifth Avenue and not a fluffy lavender taffeta thing from Goudchaux's. (No offense, Jane.)

I hired a string quartet of students from the LSU School of Music to play Christmas music as guests were arriving and as I walked down the aisle. For the reception I had a jazz band which included an elementary school piano teacher from my old neighborhood. The venue would be a remodeled plantation near St. Francisville, where my mom knew the owners and it would already be decorated for the Christmas season.

The next thing I wanted to make everything perfect was a luncheon for my bridesmaids and friends at my mom's house. I wanted to have my very own party that looked exactly like her Sunday School class Christmas party that she had been hosting for years. I wanted the card tables with red and green tablecloths and the porcelain angels surrounded by their fresh greenery. Most importantly, the giant Christmas tree in the family room and the small one in the formal living room with the complete snow village set up underneath.

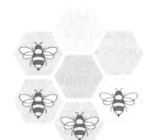

33

AFTER THAT FIRST YEAR of putting up the big tree after my father died, my mother found that her favorite local grocery store had begun selling Christmas trees. If she ordered early enough, they would not only hold an 18-foot-tall Fraser fir for her, but they would attach the stand to it, deliver it to the house, and set it up. Whew! No more ropes, sweating, and mosquito swatting.

I was in my small office in the back of my law firm's downtown building when I got a call from the owner of the grocery store that sold the Christmas trees. The man was kind and friendly, but also sounded very nervous.

"Miss Evans," he started. No one called me Miss Evans. I was Virginia. "I want you to know that we have very good insurance and will be able to pay whatever will be necessary as well as help in any way."

Insurance? Help? What was he talking about?

The store owner continued, "Well, um, you see...your mother was here to pick out a Christmas tree. You know they're all outside, in the lot behind the store, and um, well, you know it rained a lot last night, so there are several puddles in the lot. I didn't see what happened, but somehow your mother slipped and fell back there by the trees. We got her into the truck, and we've taken her to the hospital. We're with her now. Well, we asked her who we should call and she handed us your business card and asked that we contact you. They say her hip might be broken."

Ahhh. So it was starting to make sense. She hadn't memorized my work number, so she gave them my business card. "Virginia C. Evans, Attorney at Law." I guess he thought this was her way of letting him know that she was represented and that they were going to have to pay for this...so the nervousness and the insurance talk. If they only knew my mother! She would not have sued her favorite local grocery store if the owner himself had walked out and pushed her down into the puddle! She was not the litigious type, and she would not be able to show her face in that store if she sued them. No way would she be giving up Calandro's for a broken hip!

I thanked the man for taking her to the hospital and for calling me. I hung up and called Jane at her job. She was then an assistant teacher at the downtown elementary school I had attended as a child. I let her know I was leaving the office and would pick her up on the way to the hospital. This was starting to become routine.

Sure enough, my mom had a broken hip. She would have to have hip replacement surgery, followed by at least a week-long hospital stay and then physical therapy. She would be in the hospital for Thanksgiving! What were we going to do? There was so much that needed to be done. How could any of this happen without her? I needed her, didn't I?

It turns out that, before my mother fell, she had already decided on the two trees she wanted. They were delivered to her house and put up while she was in the hospital. There was so much work to be done, and she was the one who decorated the Christmas trees. But she wouldn't be able to this year. She couldn't even leave the hospital.

Molly had come to Baton Rouge from Dallas for Thanksgiving and she was a lifesaver. When I wasn't at the hospital with my mom, I was at the house with Molly frantically trying to recreate Mildred's Christmas trees. We brought lights and ornaments down from the attic. We climbed ladders and leaned over the balcony. Stringing extension cords together, we were able to get all of the lights on both trees followed by the ornaments. Then, working late into the evenings, we unpacked seemingly endless boxes of snow village houses in the living room. Using the empty boxes covered with the polyester fake snow blanket, we created hills among the village to fully display as many houses as possible. We finally had them all in place and lit up. For the first time since that addition was built, the Christmas trees were up and ready without my mother having to lift a finger. I would have my luncheon that looked like her annual Sunday School class party after all.

Once she was home from the hospital, my mom was not a good patient. She did not like the limitations put on her by her accident. She despised using her walker, insisting she could walk fine without it. I believe she quit physical therapy after merely two sessions. She was stubborn and independent. She did not like needing help, and refused it most of the times it was offered. She had missed Thanksgiving, and had to hand over her right to decorate her trees as she would have liked to. She was not happy about any of it.

I believe the day my mother broke her hip was the beginning of her transformation. My sisters and I always look back and agree that she was never quite the same after she broke her hip. She still had her feisty personality, loved her activities, her traveling, and her friends and her family. But she was different after that.

She did agree to use her walker on the night of the wedding; however, she did not give me away. My cousin, the one who made the schedule in the hospital to keep Bill and me separated, walked me down the aisle. I had all the Bees represented in the wedding party among a few friends. Katherine was maid of honor, Charlotte was a bridesmaid representing Peggy, and Elizabeth and Brittany represented Jane. They were in middle school, so I let them choose their role. Therefore, Elizabeth was the smallest bridesmaid while Brittany finally got to be a flower girl, which she had been wanting since she could walk.

Everything was beautiful, despite my sloppy amateur planning. The cake and the flowers didn't look like what I had pictured in my head that I wanted; but that was my fault and it was fine. The food and drinks were perfect, the music was fantastic, and everyone seemed to have fun. It all seemed to fly by so fast, I felt like I didn't have time to spend with hardly any of my friends. Soon the dancing was over and it was time to leave. As I bent to say goodbye to my mother, I could see how tired she was. This night had really been too much too soon for her after such a major operation. But, she wasn't going to stop or slow down for herself. She was there until the end, but I believe that evening took a further toll on her health.

34

SOMETIME BETWEEN THE ANEURYSM on her aorta and the broken hip, two other changes took place in my mom. For one, she grew shorter. This had probably been gradually happening over time, but after her brush with death she seemed smaller and weaker to me. Medically, this was caused by osteoporosis, which also contributed to the fall and the broken hip. Symbolically, it emphasized even more to me that I was the big girl now and I needed to take care of her.

The second major change was that she had to get dentures. I drove her to the procedure where the dentist pulled out all of her teeth, fitted her for the permanent dentures, and she left with temporary ones. She never got used to this. Even when the permanent dentures came in, she hated them. She claimed they hurt. I took her back to the dentist. He explained that tooth fragments were working their way out of her gums and would fall out and the dentures would feel more natural. No matter what the dentist did, the dentures never felt "natural" to her.

The dentist was young and charming. It was this that hooked my mother in. Then he would sweet-talk her through her dental appointments and, by the end of the appointment, he would somehow have her two tickets to the next LSU football game!

Seriously! These tickets had been in my family for fifty years. After my dad died, my mother did not continue the home game streak as before. She occasionally attended a game with a friend, but that was rare. But to just give them to the dentist? I was sure he was just finding things wrong as a reason for her to have to come back for a follow-up visit before each home game. Maybe he made the dentures uncomfortable on purpose. Who knows? But I didn't trust a dentist that would take football tickets from a little old lady.

And that's what she had become. A little old lady. She was shorter. She was skinnier. I think that was a result of the dentures. She never liked to eat while wearing them. It was also a result of having no one to cook a big breakfast and dinner for every night. Without doing it for someone else, what was the use of dirtying all those dishes and going to all of the trouble when you could just eat a sandwich or some cereal?

She continued to cook for the holidays and host what family was in town. Now that Jane lived next door, they began alternating. It was easier to have Christmas at Jane's house. She had small children and everyone loved watching their surprised faces as they opened their gifts. We would usually go to her house and have the gift exchange with the rustling of paper and loud squeals and laughter. It was fun no matter where it was. And Jane would have the Christmas dinner afterwards. Looking back, I don't know how she did all of that. And afterwards, without a moment to relax, she would have to round up her family and do everything all over again at her in-law's house while the rest of us went home to nap!

We may have opened gifts and eaten at Jane's, but mom still decorated her house. She still had Calandro's deliver a big tree and a little tree. Dot Debosier and I insisted she stay off of the ladder so we would decorate the top and leave the bottom for her to finish. It was so hard to get her to follow the rules. I think had she stayed with the physical therapy, kept her dentures in at all times until they felt right, and taken better care of herself, maybe she wouldn't have been so frail. But she was stubborn and would not be held back by using a walker, and she insisted she didn't need to do that physical therapy. And the trees were beautiful as usual, although I'm sure it took a lot out of her to get everything done.

She also continued to shop for everyone. We all had gifts under the tree labeled "from Santa" and still had our stockings filled by Christmas morning. I remember the Christmas Eve after she had broken her hip. It was getting late, and I was in the family room watching something on TV with Katherine when Mom looked over the balcony in a panic.

"I can't find the Harold's gift cards!" she exclaimed. Harold's was a fine clothing store that used to only be in Dallas but had recently opened a shop in Baton Rouge.

"What?" I asked.

"I bought you girls each Harold's gift cards for Christmas and I can't find them!"

"Okay, I'll come help you." For her to tell us what our gift was before Christmas meant this must be serious.

I went upstairs and began searching. "What purse were you carrying that day?" She told me and I began going through all the contents of the bag. Then I checked her other purses. I looked around her room and then downstairs in the junk drawer under the microwave. As we searched, she became more and more agitated. She began to act desperate. She was so upset. I don't believe it had to do with the potentially lost money, but the fact she couldn't remember where she had "hidden" the cards.

I finally gave up searching. "Mom, I have a friend who works there. I will go talk to her the day after Christmas and see if they can be replaced."

She seemed somewhat relieved, but we could tell she was still upset.

Now, I've hidden things from my girls and forgotten where they were. I've purchased the perfect birthday card for a sister well in advance and then run out to buy her a card the day before her birthday, completely forgetting that I already had the perfect card...in my junk drawer. And I'm much younger than my mom was at the age when she misplaced the gift cards.

Was something in her worried about not remembering? Did she sense a problem? If so, she was not going to admit it to anyone. I had the gift cards canceled and reissued the day after Christmas as promised. And, a few months later, when my mom came

across the original gift cards, we simply cut them up and threw
them away, forgetting the incident about forgetting.

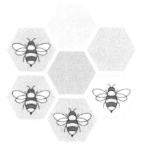

35

AFTER MY DAD DIED, my mom took on the yard work. This meant she drove the riding lawn mower over the acre or more of grass that surrounded our house. She did not use the weedeater or the blower—just the lawn mower. Soon, the rectangular marble pavers that led from the driveway to the front door were so overgrown with grass that they could no longer be seen. Bushes in the front exploded in disarray. Vines that were never there before climbed the redwood siding, some even sneaking through cracks between the windows and their frames to see what it was like to grow inside.

Inside the house began to grow disorderly. Slowly, not overnight. My mom stopped throwing anything away. The kitchen table and counter became cluttered with junk mail and bills. Catalogues and newspapers piled up all over the house. And then she found the letters.

When the houses were separated and Jane moved into the old part, she was helping to empty everything and move Mom's things next door. While checking a rarely used deep cabinet above the built-in chest of drawers and closet in what used to be her bedroom, she discovered a wooden box. When she opened the box, she realized it contained the letters my parents had written to each other during World War II. Neatly organized by number, in chronological order, they had been pristinely stored for more than fifty years. This level of organization was obviously done by my dad.

What had once been my dad's drawing room, now with carpet and walls, had become a makeshift spare bedroom, but mostly a junk depository. There was now a twin bed in case an extra bed was needed for out-of-town company. My mom's desk from the downtown office was set up in there as well. On it sat my first computer from while I was in law school. This thing would be a dinosaur now, but it had Windows and WordPerfect and a *slooooooowwwww* dial-up modem for online research, so it did what I needed it to do. The rest of the room was mostly covered in boxes of various papers and artifacts which had been moved from the downtown office, but never unpacked. Now that Jane was moving next door, it also contained things from the old house that didn't have a place to go yet my mom was not ready to throw away.

It was in this room that the box of letters was placed during the move. But they would not stay in that box, nor would they stay in order for very long.

Like I said, my mother was never the same after she broke her hip. She still went to Pace's every Thursday morning and had her hair done. She had a regular Thursday bridge game at alternating houses or, occasionally, at a private room at Juban's, a local restaurant. On Fridays, she volunteered as a docent at the LSU alumni center, greeting visitors, answering their questions and directing them as to where to go. And she occasionally traveled with either Dot Debosier or Dot Howell.

She had traded in her large Chrysler New Yorker for a smaller Chrysler sedan, and they used this car to visit Uncle Charlie on occasion. After a day of eating his rich food and listening to his entertaining stories, she would always purchase several large coolers full of fresh gulf shrimp to take home to Baton Rouge. It was on one of these trips in her new car that one of the coolers leaked. New car smell gone, dead shrimp smell in. It was awful. Impossible to clean out or cover up. I took it to professionals and had it detailed. I sprinkled baking soda all over it and vacuumed it later. I sprayed Febreze. But, despite my efforts, the new car always had a slight stench of dead shrimp.

On the rest of her days, without having to run my dad's office or prepare meals for anyone, she became idle. I stopped by often to visit her. She could be found at the kitchen table, playing solitaire on a clean area away from which she had swiped away the clutter of mail. I would also find her in bed. Covered in the letters. That's right. In her idle time, she was reliving her young romance by reading and rereading every letter ever written between my father and her. Sometimes, I would even find her on the small twin bed in the old drawing room covered in letters. As she read and descended into her memories, she became covered in the clutter of new and old mail. I believe that is when this clutter began to spread to her mind.

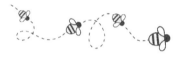

Around this time, I left my first law firm to go out on my own. At first, I had a partner, then I ran the business by myself. It was a title company. I finally took the knowledge I had learned from the mortgage company in Dallas and was using it in combination with my law degree.

One of the things I hated about being on my own was marketing. It's not like I thought I could just hang up a sign and clients would start flooding into my office; however, I didn't realize how hard it would be to convince clients to use me instead of someone else as their title attorney.

I began baking these chocolate chip bundt cakes sprinkled with powdered sugar. Jane had given me the recipe years before. The cakes were not only melt-in-your-mouth delicious, but they looked pretty. I then went to party stores and bought as many square cake boxes as they sold.

I would mix, pour, bake, and sprinkle all day and into the night. I bought more pans so I had an assembly line going in my kitchen. After the cakes had cooled, I placed them in the boxes I had purchased and tied them with ribbons and a big bow. Finally, I attached my business card to the cake box.

The day after a night of baking and boxing, I would drive around Baton Rouge to different banks, mortgage companies, and Realtor offices, delivering my cakes. If someone was there to listen to me, I would talk about my firm and my mortgage and legal experience. Then I would return home and resume baking to deliver to more potential contacts the next day.

The big title companies hired marketing personnel whose entire job was to keep the lenders and realtors happy and keep their name in front of them. I was starting out and couldn't afford such a person, so it was up to me. When someone asked me my position with the company, I would always reply, "Lawyer, secretary, janitor, marketing executive, accountant, maid..."

Fortunately, my client base began to build. I'm not sure if the cakes had anything to do with it. I provided personal service that larger firms couldn't offer. My clients appreciated this and continued to refer real estate closings to me.

By now, the interest rates were going down again, much lower than the rates when I was in Dallas. People were not only buying homes, but they were refinancing their 8.5% mortgages for loans with 6% interest. So business was coming in, the bills were being paid, and though I was busy, I also had the freedom that came with working for myself. I loved the faces of first-time home buyers after they had signed all their documents and were handed the keys to their new homes. I was performing a service that was on the happier side of practicing law and I was being paid to do something I actually enjoyed.

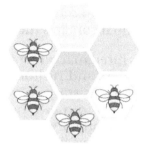

36

THE CHANGE IN MY mom was slow. It was subtle. She had been telling the same stories over and over for years, either not remembering that she had already told it or maybe thinking it was worth retelling. Many of these stories stick in my head to this day.

By now Katherine had been dating Cotty since 1993, the summer my dad died. Cotty's full name is Carleton A. Jones III. He is from Johnson City, Tennessee, and he was the center on the high school football team when Steve Spurrier was the quarterback. They remain friends to this day and Cotty has followed Florida, Washington, and later South Carolina football to cheer on his friend, "The Head Ball Coach."

One of the stories my mom always told and retold went like this: When she served as the alumni representative on the LSU Athletic Council and they were interviewing for a new head football coach to replace Bill Arnsparger in 1987, she had a chance to participate in Steve Spurrier's (then head football coach at Duke) interview for the job. She loved to tell that everyone just oohed and aahed over him until she asked him the question, "If the head coaching position at Florida should become open while you are working at LSU, would you leave

LSU for Florida?" I can't remember if she claimed he didn't answer or he answered yes, anyway, she swore her question was why LSU did not hire Steve Spurrier that year. Thanks a lot Mom, for Mike Archer, and the beginning of a decade of losing!

Now Katherine and Cotty have mentioned this to Steve Spurrier, who denies remembering or answering any such question, but my mom argued to anyone who would listen that this was the absolute truth. And no one could convince her otherwise.

That was just one of the stories told and retold. She often talked about how ever since the day her daddy got killed, she and Charlie had to go to work and give all their money to her Mama! That bit of resentment stayed with her and was repeated for most of her life.

But now she was repeating things she had just recently said. Or asking questions that she had already asked only moments before. It was best just to go along with it and not argue with her. If you told her she already said it, it would just start an argument and it wasn't worth it. She still had enough wits about her to remember how my Mawmaw was at the end, and she continued to warn us that, "If I ever get like that, just lock me up in a nursing home and forget about me! I mean it! And don't even visit!"

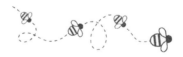

Around this time, we decided to have a birthday party for my mom at my house. I had recently moved from a rented duplex and purchased a small home. We had a fenced-in yard and a nice deck, as well as a relatively large kitchen for a home of that size. Since her birthday was in April, we decided it would be a crawfish boil. That's the best kind of party in the spring down here. Everything is blooming, the weather is not too hot yet, and cooking and eating outside feels magnificent. The spices from the boiling pot can clear your sinuses. Then the hot, red crawfish along with corn, potatoes, and anything else the cook cares to boil, are dumped on a table covered in newspaper. Everyone stands around the table enjoying cold beer while peeling and eating the spicy crustaceans and sides.

Jane and her family came over as well as my cousin, Cecil. Peggy had come into town and rode in the car with my mother to the party at my house. I remember the weather was much hotter than usual for mid-April, so it wasn't quite as comfortable outside as I would have preferred, but the food and drinks were great, followed by singing, candles, and birthday cake. One by one, full and satisfied, guests began to leave. I was still drinking and talking in my backyard when Cecil approached me. He said, "I don't know if you want to hear this right now, but I just watched your mother drive away with Peggy, and she just ran over all of your azalea bushes."

"What?" I ran to the front yard to check the damage. The bushes were turned somewhat on their sides, but they were old and established and would survive. The marks from the tires showed that the small Chrysler sedan had indeed straddled the azaleas when leaving the house.

Oh no, I thought. *This can't happen. She HAS to be able to drive! If she can't, she will be miserable. It will be the end of her.*

I told him I understood it was a problem and reported the incident to the Bees. We all took it pretty lightly, laughing about it along with the Spurrier story and the Harold's gift cards. "She's going crazy," we would joke. Thinking of it as real or serious was too much for any of us to handle yet. She was just acting funny or silly, like when a small child says something wrong but in a way that makes everyone laugh.

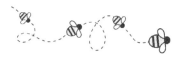

After several visits to my mom's house and observing the clutter everywhere, I began to go through the mail that had been scattered all over the kitchen. To my surprise, she had accumulated a large amount of credit card debt on which she had made no payments. She not only had unpaid bills, but letters from collection agencies.

"Mom, when did you get all these credit cards? And what did you buy?" I didn't see anything new around the house.

"I don't know why they keep sending that junk to me," she casually replied, "I don't even have any credit cards."

"Well, these companies seem to think you do. Are you absolutely sure?"

"Yes, I'm absolutely sure. I don't have a single credit card from any of those people and I don't understand why they keep sending those bills."

"Okay, let me take them with me and look into it."

"Sure, if you want to. But you don't have to because they're not mine."

I collected the bills and letters and brought them to my office. The next day, I began contacting the companies to get information about the debts. I started out by stating that I was Mrs. Evans' attorney and that she did not have these credit cards. I was aggressive, demanding information. A mistake had been made and now they were harassing my mom instead of the real debtor.

I soon discovered what I believe to be an abhorrent scheme used by creditors which can easily confuse both elderly and younger folks as well. The bank or credit card company would send a check made payable to the addressee for an obscure amount, such as $8,425.36. Not a neat round number. The check would be attached by perforation to a letter which, in very fine print, stated that this was a pre-approved loan and that, if cashed, the addressee agrees to pay back the full amount in monthly installments at an exorbitant rate of interest.

It seems my mother, without reading anything on the attachments, had been either cashing or depositing these checks. I demanded proof and when I received the fax of the front and back of the check, it was clear to me that the checks had been endorsed in my mother's beautiful and unmistakable cursive. I would recognize that signature and handwriting anywhere. It was hers. But what had she done with the money?!

I went back to her house and explained the situation to her. She claimed not to know about cashing any checks that would be considered loans and maintained that she did not owe anyone. The debts added up to over $60,000 and with her Social Security money and my dad's army retirement, if she made the minimum payments every month, the debts would not be paid off for ages. I knew it was time for something to be done. I needed to start protecting her.

Since I owned a title company, I had several banking contacts. I called a banker client of mine and applied for a home equity loan on my mother's behalf. This was approved and the money would be used to pay off the credit card debt. Reading the history of the title to that home was remarkable to me.

My parents had purchased the lot for $11,000. They had borrowed very little to build the home and there hadn't been a mortgage on it for decades. The neighborhood had grown in its prestige as Baton Rouge had spread out, having more and more new subdivisions, and large lots with mature trees became more rare. So even with a $60,000 mortgage, my mom would still have substantial equity in her house.

The next step was to have her sign a power of attorney to me. I assured her that I was in no way trying to control her and that she would still have her checkbook and access to her money. I just needed a way to protect her, and without a power of attorney, banks would not let me deal with them on her behalf. She finally agreed and signed the document.

After going to the bank and having my name added to her account, I took up the task of sending letters to every creditor I could find in the stacks of mail I recovered from her house. I sent every predator, as I felt they were, a copy of the power of attorney and notice that she lacked capacity to enter into any contracts and that nothing signed solely by her would be considered valid. I hoped I had done enough. She obviously needed protecting.

We still have no idea where the money went from all those checks she cashed. Believe me, we looked everywhere. We never noticed any newly purchased, expensive items in the house. Hopefully, one day the mystery of the predator creditor money will finally be solved.

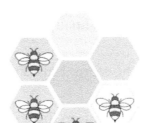

37

WITH THE CLUTTER, DEBTS, and bad driving, we were beginning to realize Mom wasn't improving. While she was still driving her car, Jane's husband had been taking over driving the riding lawn mower. She still dressed up for her hair appointment and bridge every Thursday and for the LSU Alumni Center every Friday.

The holidays were still important to her and she continued to decorate her house. She loved stuffed bunnies and placed them all around her house at Easter time along with the delicate eggs, chicks, and other springtime paraphernalia. Once, when her birthday was before Easter, Jane and I went in together and bought her a very nice and fairly expensive stuffed bunny. It was handmade and every detail was precious. Ears, nose, whiskers, paws, I can see it now being placed out for display every Easter. Except it wasn't.

Brittany's birthday is also in April, before my mom's. The following year, Jane held a party for Brittany at her house next door to my mom. I parked at Mom's and walked with her to the party, each of us carrying our gift for Brittany. When Brittany opened the gift from my mom, imagine how Jane and I felt when it was the exact bunny we had picked out and given Mom the year before!

Not only did she regift the present we so carefully thought about to give her, she had some elaborate story to go with it. She told everyone about how she knew how much Brittany loved bunnies (actually, Brittany has always favored giraffes). Then she told how she shopped everywhere and finally, at this nice gift shop, found this bunny.

"Oh, when I saw it in the store, I just knew I had to buy it for Brittany!"

Jane and I had to bite our bottom lips to keep from laughing in front of everyone. She really believed every word she was saying. And just like hearing the same stories over and over, it was easier to just let her go on believing it. Everyone was realizing that she was beginning to live in her own little imaginary world and, though she would return to ours every now and then, we weren't going into hers.

Her nutrition and hygiene began to deteriorate. She had always been the greatest cook I had ever known, but I now did not trust any food she prepared. Once I walked into the kitchen for a visit and she was standing over the stove stirring something in her black iron skillet. I had tasted so many wonderful recipes of hers, many of which started in this very skillet. But this looked unfamiliar. It was an unrecognizable, mushy, mixture which she continued to somewhat sauté. As she pushed the glob back and forth, I asked her what she was making.

"Ghoulash," she replied.

"Ghoulash? What in the world is that?"

"Oh hush! You know what that is. I always make that!"

What I was looking at somewhat resembled sautéed canned dog food and was not something I had ever heard of or seen her make before. Happy to have a visitor, she pushed the skillet to the back burner and sat down at the kitchen table to talk. I walked over and turned off the stove before sitting down with her.

She was also becoming incontinent. I tried my best to ignore it at first. They say smells evoke more memories than any of the other senses. She was beginning to smell like MawMaw, and I did not like the mental pictures that came to mind when I thought of that. Her blue La-Z-Boy chair, where Bill sat to eat ice cream, was soaking up the smell. So was her car. I knew it was real when

I noticed that the shrimp smell was gone. None of that cleaning could get rid of it. But with a good dose of stale urine smell, the odor of dead shrimp vanished forever.

My sisters noticed all these things, too. We got together and told stories of what crazy things Mom had been doing. Sitting around, sipping beer or wine, repeating:

"I mean, she REALLY thought she bought that bunny for Brittany! She made up a whole shopping story about it!"

"Well, at least she didn't drive over your azalea bushes!"

"If she tells that Steve Spurrier story to Cotty one more time, I'm going to lose it!"

"Remember when her mom was like that? All she used to say was, 'If I ever get like that, lock me up in a nursing home and forget about me! Don't even visit!'"

"The problem is, when you get like that, you don't think you're doing anything wrong, so that doesn't work."

And on and on. Repeating what Mom had been doing. Not wanting to do anything about it. So we just went on talking and laughing.

38

On the morning of September 11, 2001, I was still in bed when Katherine called me.

"Are you watching TV?" she asked. She's an hour ahead of me so she doesn't always realize how early it is for me. It was a Tuesday, though, so I needed to get up and start getting ready for work anyway.

"No, I'm just waking up. Why?"

"An airplane hit the World Trade Center."

"Aww, man! Was anybody hurt? How did it happen? What kind of plane?" Like a lot of people, we thought it must have been an accident. A small private plane that had lost control.

"I'm not sure. I feel so sorry for the people in that plane. I wonder if it hit anyone in the building?"

"I'm going to get some coffee and go watch it. I'll call you later." I went to the kitchen to make my morning coffee. I usually just shower and go to work without watching TV in the morning, but since she had made a point to call me about it, I decided to turn it on.

By now it was clear that it was a commercial airline full of people and that it had crashed into the building and exploded. I called her back.

"Oh my God! Can you imagine being in that building? Or on that plane? I wonder what happened to it?"

Another plane flew into the second tower and exploded. America was under attack. Katherine and I stayed on the phone all morning. Occasionally taking a break and hanging up. Then another crash, and one of us would call back. The towers were burning, people in the floors above the crash were jumping to their deaths to avoid burning. All commercial airlines were ordered to land.

"Can you imagine if one of those buildings fell down?" Katherine asked.

"It's weird, but I just recently watched a show on Discovery or some channel like that about how those towers were built. The engineering is really remarkable. There's no way they could actually..." My voice trailed off as I watched the tower begin its descent into a massive cloud of dust that traveled and covered people with debris for blocks.

We talked and cried as we watched the second tower fall, the Pentagon burn, and the remains of the plane that went down in Pennsylvania. My Kennedy assassination day was here. I would always remember where I was and what I was doing when I heard about the terror attacks on September 11.

All flights in the United States had been ordered grounded and no planes would be taking off again for days as the country was still shocked and confused.

On this day, my mom happened to be on one of her gambling trips with Dot Debosier. This one was not on the Mississippi Gulf Coast. This time they had actually gone to Las Vegas! I had been excited for her to be going on this trip, but now I was worried because she was stuck there with no plane to fly her home.

I received a call from Dot Debosier on the afternoon of Thursday, September 13 that they had finally been able to fly home and that my mother was at her house. I immediately drove over to visit her. What I found became the beginning of the end.

Once I arrived, I entered the back door looking for her to be playing solitaire on the kitchen table. The house was getting darker as evening approached and was eerily quiet. I took the stairs two at a time to get to my mom's bedroom. She was lying in bed, awake but silent.

"Oh my God, Mom! I'm so glad you're home and safe. Are you okay?"

"Of course I'm okay. Why wouldn't I be?"

"I was just so worried when they grounded all the planes. I didn't know when you would get home or how. I guess I'm just relieved."

"What do you mean, 'grounded all the planes'? What are you talking about?"

"The terror attacks on Tuesday! Weren't you afraid? I've been so upset ever since then."

"What attacks? I'm fine!"

Just then the phone rang. I answered the extension next to my mom's bed and heard Dot Debosier's voice, "Virginia?"

"Yes."

"I think I need to talk to you about your mother."

"Okay."

"Do you think I need to talk to you about your mother?"

"Yes. Should I come over now?"

"Yes," and she hung up.

I told my mom I would be right back and walked next door to the Debosiers' house. My mom had been forgetting things. And maybe not as clean and elegant as she once was. But this was different. How could she not know about the largest attack on the United States since Pearl Harbor? One that targeted civilians and changed everything? What was going on?

As I entered the Debosiers' house, Dot Debosier sat me down at her kitchen table.

"Your mom is sick. You know that, right?"

"Yes. She's been forgetful in the past, but to not know about 9/11? How could that be?"

"It's not just that. It was a bad trip for her. She was found by security wandering around the casino barefoot in her nightgown. She had no idea who she was with or where she was. They were somehow able to connect her to me. I was able to get her to the room and dressed. But then the flights were grounded and we had to stay two extra days. I have had to watch her at all times. She didn't know where she was or what had happened, even with the news on TV 24/7."

I began tearing up. How was I going to handle this?!

"There's one more thing," she said, "Your mom is the one who drove us home from the airport in her car. She drove on sidewalks, stopped for no reason, missed turns, it was awful. I just knew we were going to die or kill someone else in that car."

"Okay, I'll handle it." I said as I closed the door and slowly returned to my mom.

She was still in bed. She seemed exhausted, I guess that was from traveling.

"What are you doing here?"

"Oh nothing. I was just checking on you to see if you enjoyed your trip."

"What trip?"

"Never mind. Do you need anything before I leave?"

"No."

"Okay. I'll come back to see you real soon."

Before I left, I discreetly gathered every key to her car and placed them in my purse. I wasn't sure what I would do next, but I could not let her behind the wheel of a vehicle ever again.

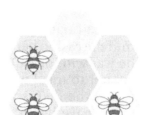

39

I SOBBED THE WHOLE drive back to my house. My mind was still processing the attack on our country, the loss of lives, the heroes who went up into the buildings while everyone else was exiting. I had been glued to the news and the stories of tragedy and heroism, the voicemails left by loved ones prior to their impending death, the images of people jumping out of buildings, and the survivors found under the rubble.

Now I had to add this to my list to be sad about. My mom had gone from forgetful and bad driver to seemingly full-on dementia and dangerous driver in a matter of days. I knew I had to do something and it had to be done fast. She was now a danger to herself and possibly others.

I immediately called my sisters and reported what had happened. Everyone agreed something needed to be done, but no one quite knew what. The next morning, I decided it was time for me to act. I was now going to be the caregiver to the woman who not only gave me life, but took care of me in every way for all of it up to that point.

My first call the next day was to her doctor's office, the same primary care physician who had been seeing my dad. When my parents had begun seeing him, their old family physician, who also sat behind them in Tiger Stadium, had retired. At first, they were treated as well as they had always been. But as health insurance, HMOs, PPOs, and new government regulations grew, the doctor's office became less and less personal.

When I made the call, I was asked the nature of the problem and told that the nurse would call me back. Several hours later, I received the call from his nurse.

"What seems to be wrong with Mrs. Evans?"

"She went away on a vacation over 9/11 and, once she was home, she was different. She barely remembers anything. She's not talking as much. Something is definitely wrong and she needs to see the doctor."

"Well, he can see her in two weeks. Will that work?"

"No! Something is really wrong! She needs to see him today."

"If you believe she's had a stroke, you need to take her to the emergency room."

My frustration with this woman and this whole office was building.

"She needs to see Dr. Parker. He knows her! He will be able to tell the difference. I don't think it's a stroke and I don't think an emergency room is the right place for her."

"Well, his first available appointment for a physical checkup is in two weeks."

"No! She doesn't need a routine physical. Something has happened to her. Something is wrong. She needs to see him and it needs to be today."

"Okay, let me talk to him and I will call you back."

"Thank you." I hung up the phone, both pissed off and relieved. Why do they have to give everyone the runaround? Why can't you just call your doctor and talk to him? This leaving messages and waiting was driving me crazy. What in the world was I supposed to do? I needed a doctor to tell me what to do, and how to take care of my mother.

I tried to work despite the distractions. Wanting to keep my eyes on the news. Wanting the doctor's office to call back. I couldn't focus on anything at my office. There wasn't very much work to do anyway. People weren't out trying to buy or refinance a house in those weeks following 9/11. I believe everyone was glued to the images on the TV screens, still in shock, still mourning.

The nurse finally called back and said that the doctor would see my mother that afternoon. I left the office and drove to her house to get her up and dressed. She didn't understand why I thought she needed a doctor, but complied peacefully and went along with me.

After what seemed like hours in the waiting room, followed by waiting in the examination room, the doctor finally entered.

"So, Mildred, how are you today?"

"I'm fine. I don't even know why I'm here."

"Well, Virginia here is a little concerned about you, so I'm just going to ask you a few questions."

"Okay."

"Do you remember what happened on Tuesday?"

"Of course I do, why wouldn't I?"

"How do you feel about the attacks?"

"What attacks?"

"On the World Trade Center and the Pentagon."

"Oh, did somebody try to set off a bomb again?" She said, so nonchalantly.

"Hmm. I'm going to tell you three words and I want you to repeat them to me."

"Alright."

"Elephant, radio, bicycle."

"Elephant, radio, bicycle," she repeated, back straight, shoulders back, proud of herself.

"Now, I'm going to examine you and we're going to talk some more, then I want you to tell me those three words again."

"Fine."

He began to listen to her heart. He took out his light and looked into her eyes, ears, nose, and throat. He listened to her chest as he asked her to take deep breaths. He talked about LSU football and how everyone was wondering when LSU would get to play Auburn, now that the game had been postponed due to 9/11. After about ten minutes of examination and chitchat, he asked her to repeat the three words he had told her earlier.

"What three words?" she asked.

"Earlier, when I asked you to repeat three words to me. What were those three words?"

"You didn't ask me to repeat three words. I don't know what you're talking about. Why am I here? I'm not sick."

"You're right, you're fine. I'm going to step outside with Virginia and you just relax for a few minutes, okay?"

He held the door open for me as we stepped out into the hall.

"Well, she's right about one thing. She's not physically sick. There's nothing I can do about her condition today. She will need to see a neurologist. I will have my nurse call and make the appointment for you. It usually takes a few weeks to get in."

"Weeks! But what am I supposed to do with her in the meantime?"

"She's not still living in her house alone is she?"

"Yes."

"Well, that's too dangerous for her. She'll either need sitters or you'll need to place her in a facility."

Facility. A nursing home? *"If I ever get like that, I want you all to just lock me up in a nursing home and forget about me! Don't even visit."* Her old words kept haunting my brain.

"Her neighbor told me she drove yesterday and she was driving on the sidewalk and all over the place. She was scared to death."

"She absolutely cannot drive anymore."

I knew this. I had already taken away all the keys to her car. But who was going to tell her this? Not driving would devastate her. It would strip away all her independence. What about getting her hair done? Playing bridge? The alumni center?

"Can you tell her that?"

"Yes, I will tell her, but you're going to have to enforce it. No driving. And start finding a safe place for her to live."

We walked back into the examining room, where my mom sat waiting, unconcerned, convinced nothing was wrong with her.

"Now Mildred, I've told Virginia this and now I'm going to tell you. I am ordering that you not drive anymore."

"What?! Why? I can drive!" Now she was getting mad.

"I am writing this down on my prescription pad and I am going to hand it to you. Whenever you even think about driving, I want you to look at this piece of paper and know that you are under doctor's orders to stop driving."

"For how long?"

"Until I say you can. For now, you are no longer allowed to drive," he admonished her as he handed her the prescription slip. I glanced at it and it read, "Mildred Evans is not to drive a car per doctor's order." It was signed and dated by him.

"You can go now. Virginia is going to take you to another doctor to get you further checked out. Good luck. I'll see you soon." Then looking at me, he added, "You will need to start bringing her in regularly to check her Coumadin levels so that we can adjust the dosage."

So this was it. I would be taking her to the doctor. She wouldn't be driving. She wouldn't be getting better. I had so many questions running through my head. Questions about my mother and about our country. What had started out as a nice fall week, looking forward to a home LSU game on Saturday, had turned into one of the worst weeks for my life and the life of the world.

40

I CAME HOME AND called my sisters. It soon became clear to us that something had to be done. Well, several things had to be done to take care of my mother. It was also clear that none of this would happen fast. There was no urgency from the doctor. There was no emergency room that could make this better. It was going to be a long process. And we had no idea what we were doing.

Our roles soon began to define themselves. As the lawyer in the family, and the one with Mom's power of attorney, I would be handling her finances and legal decisions. Jane was next door, so she would check on Mom periodically, making sure she was safe, fed, cleaned, and taking her medicine. Peggy and Katherine would come to Baton Rouge as often as they could to help out. Once in town, they would drive to any appointments or places Mom needed to be, and they would stay with her and take care of her needs at home.

I did not bring up the driving issue with my mom on the way home from the doctor or at any other time, but she finally caught on that I was in between her and her car, and she wanted me out of the way. She called early the following week in an outrage.

"I have looked all over this house and I cannot find the keys to my car!"

"I know, Mom. Remember, the doctor said you are not allowed to drive."

"Which doctor? When?"

"Look in your purse. You will find a prescription from the doctor stating that you are not allowed to drive. I had to take your keys away so that you wouldn't drive. It is not safe for you or other people for you to be driving right now."

"Why not? I'm not sick. There's nothing wrong with me." She was becoming desperate. She was not going to take this lightly.

"Mom, when you need to go somewhere, let me or Jane know, and we can take you."

"I need to be able to drive myself! What about my hair appointment? I have things I need to do. I need groceries. Bring those keys back to my house now! You cannot tell me what to do and you have no right to take my keys!" She was full-blown angry now. And I was sad. Not the kind of sad I would be as a child if she were angry at me for some misbehavior. I was sad because she was angry at me and I was not going to be able to make it better. I could not endanger lives just to have her not be angry at me. But it hurt me deep inside. I had always tried to be the people pleaser, the one who made my parents laugh, or made them proud. My worst nightmare was to make them mad at me. And now I had done it. But it had to be done. And, no matter how much I wanted her to like me, I could not back down.

Knowing that the doctor would back me up and would never authorize her to drive again, I tried one more tactic.

"Okay, Mom. The doctor says you are not supposed to drive. It says so on the prescription. I will pick you up tomorrow morning and take you to get your hair done and any errands you need to go on. We will make sure you get rides to bridge, the alumni center, any place you need to go. But until the doctor personally calls me and tells me that you are allowed to drive, I will not be giving you back your keys."

"Fine, then. Don't be late in the morning. I need to be at Pace's by 8:00." And with that, she ended the call.

The following morning became the first ride to Pace's that I would end up making every Thursday for years. It was awful. I had to get up and get ready before my usual time, then drive across town to get her, back to Pace's, wait, then take her back home, then go to work. It was particularly inconvenient because while Pace's was less than a five minute drive from my house, it was about fifteen to twenty minutes from my mom's house.

As I walked in that first day of dropping her off, I was immediately hit by years of memories. Nothing had changed. We parted the strings of wooden beads to get through the doors. The big orange round chairs that I used to spin around in were still in the waiting area, and all of the smells were exactly the same as if I had been five years old. And the same people were there. Janice, who cut my hair as a child, was still there "doing" Mom's hair every Thursday morning. And Mom knew all the people who had appointments on those mornings. That's where she got her real news about what was going on in Baton Rouge, and she was not going to miss out on it.

She turned around and dismissed me. I'm sure she was embarrassed and didn't want to explain why I was dropping her off. I think all the ladies in there had been expecting this, and I seemed to detect a hint of relief that my mother would not be behind the wheel on any public roads. I lived close enough to go back to my house and wait until she was finished before picking her up and driving her home.

Eventually, I figured out how to time it where I could jump out of bed, grab a coffee, pick up mom, drive her to Pace's, then go back to my house to shower and get dressed for work. That trimmed a little of the wasted time off and made it somewhat more peaceful, even though I still dreaded every Thursday morning.

I also figured out it was a much more pleasant ride if I brought along my Golden Retriever, Ella. Golden Retrievers have one of the best smiles of any dog breed, and Ella's was no different. It was hard to be sad around that dog. As I drove to pick up my mom, I would look at Ella smiling from the backseat. Usually I would play "Your Smiling Face" by James Taylor on the way. Truly, every time I saw her smiling face, I had to smile myself. Mom enjoyed having Ella in the car, too. With her seatbelt on, she would ride almost the entire time turned around, looking and smiling at that dog for the entire ride. So, despite the drawbacks of this weekly errand, I at least found some ways to lighten up the ride and not start my day off entirely grumpy.

Of course, even with her hair done, Mom still had plenty of other places she needed to be. Friends volunteered to take her to her weekly bridge games, and to the LSU Alumni Center, where she still served as a docent on Friday mornings. But Jane and I had the rest, which consisted mostly of grocery trips and doctor visits.

The first time I took her to the neurologist, she was extremely confused. It was not her normal doctor's office and, since she still maintained that nothing was wrong with her, she felt she did not need to be there. They called our name and we were shown to an examination room. The neurologist who entered was a large, kind woman with a gentle nature. Her voice was soothing, not rough like the family doctor.

"Good afternoon, Mrs. Evans, it's so nice to meet you."

"It's nice to meet you, too. But I don't know why I'm here."

"Well, let's just talk for a while and get to know one another."

"Alright with me."

The doctor then proceeded to ask my mom a series of questions, which I recognized as a test. Just like the family doctor, she had her repeat three words and she promptly complied. Once again, she did not remember the three words five minutes later. She was asked who was the president and other general knowledge questions that she should have known. The doctor also examined her physically and performed several coordination tests. Soon she asked me to step outside, leaving my mom alone in the examination room.

"She definitely has dementia," she began, "This can be caused by a series of mini strokes in her brain, which is entirely possible given her history of blood clots. Or it could be Alzheimer's disease. I will need to order an MRI of her brain to determine the cause and the course of treatment."

"Treatment? There's a treatment?" I had given up hope.

"Well, there are medications that can slow the progression of the disease; however, there is no cure."

My heart felt heavy. I hadn't had much hope, but just that one spark was already burning out. She gave me a prescription for Xanax to give to my mother to relax her for the MRI, which I scheduled on the way out of the office.

Later, I took my mother to the MRI, relaxed from the pill she had taken. Once the results were in, we were back in the neurologist's office and I was in the hall with the doctor while my mom was alone in the examining room.

"The results have shown that your mother does have Alzheimer's disease."

I was not surprised, but that didn't stop me from being disappointed. "So what do we do now?"

"I'm going to prescribe a medicine called Aricept. It may slow the progression of the disease. However, your mother's condition seems to be more advanced than when most people start this medication. I do believe it is worth a try. I am also going to prescribe Zoloft to help with her mood. Unlike patients with mini strokes, Alzheimer's patients tend to get extremely irritable."

I thought about her anger when I took the keys. "Yes, thank you. She needs the Zoloft."

"You also need to get her some home care or move her to a facility. It is no longer safe for her to live alone at home."

"I know." I thought of her in her bed in the house where she had lived for half a century. Covering herself in the letters written by my dad, and her letters to him. How could she leave this place? I knew it was going to be a fight beyond any comparison to the fight about driving and I decided this was not the day to start. I scheduled a follow-up appointment and took my mother home. Home...how could I make her leave this place?

"If I ever get like that, just lock me up in a nursing home and forget about me!" Her words, which had come back to me so many times since my grandmother was sick, seemed so simple. What I never knew back then when she said those words to us is that, by the time you "get like that," you don't believe anything is wrong with you and you fight anyone who accuses you of being "like that." This was going to suck!

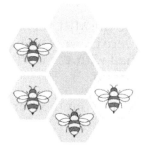

41

FOR THE NEXT FEW months, we went along as usual. I drove to the hair appointment every Thursday morning, with Ella in the backseat. Jane made sure Mom was eating, taking her medicine, and staying safe. We took turns with the other errands. And all four of us discussed what to do about her living situation.

Once, I called her to let her know I would be coming by to take her grocery shopping. She said okay and was dressed and ready to go when I walked in the back door. I glanced down at her hand and noticed a piece of paper gripped strongly in her fingers.

"What do you have there?"

"My shopping list."

"Oh great! That will be a big help. Can I see it?"

I took the paper from her and turned it over. On the back side of a used envelope she had scribbled out a list.

Cereal
Bread
Coffee
Milk
Bathroom tissue
Soup
Anything I see that I want or can use

This final item made me laugh and melted my heart at the same time. I had been noticing that she was forgetful. Even irritable. But then it dawned on me that she was also becoming childlike. Her innocence was so sweet. She began surrounding herself with stuffed animals from around the house. She got excited about the simplest things. Like a sweet, innocent child. Except when she wasn't.

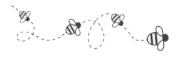

The nurse from Dr. Parker's office called me at work one afternoon. Hmmm...they never called me; they barely answered when I tried to call them. I answered and asked what I could do for her.

"It's your mom. I don't understand what she's talking about and I don't know what to do."

Talking about? Mom didn't have an appointment that day. What was she doing now?

"She's been calling all day long. Each time I talk to her, she demands that Dr. Parker call you and tell you that she can drive again. He can't do that, but she won't stop calling. I thought he made it clear she couldn't drive anymore."

Then I remembered. In order to calm her down about the driving, I had shown her the doctor's note on the prescription pad and said the only way I would give her back the keys was if Dr. Parker called me and told me it was okay. Now she couldn't remember three words from five minutes ago, but she certainly remembered what I said about her driving. Was this whole memory thing selective?

"I'm so sorry. I was just trying to calm her down and told her she couldn't drive unless Dr. Parker called me to say it was okay. It honestly never occurred to me that she would remember that or start bothering you. Just keep telling her no. I'll take care of the car."

I went home wondering what in the world I was going to do. I had taken the keys, but the car was still sitting in Mom's carport, tempting her. It was time to get rid of it and I just knew she would hate me for it. The idea of not driving made her so angry she could spit nails. And I was the target of that anger. As much as it hurt to have her mad at me, I knew I was saving lives by keeping her off of the streets...and sidewalks, and azalea bushes.

The next time I visited my mom it was as if her neighbor had been watching and waiting for me to visit. Mom's phone rang as I came in the back door and I walked to the counter by the stove to answer it.

"Virginia," Dot Debosier started, "what are you planning to do with your mother's car?"

"I was just wondering that myself."

"Well, I would like to buy it if you don't mind. I will give you $10,000 for it."

I didn't have any idea what the car was worth. It was relatively new with very low mileage. But it had that smell. I knew Dot had ridden in it recently, so she either didn't mind the smell of stale pee and dead shrimp, or her sense of smell was failing her. Regardless, I wasn't interested in trying to sell that car on my own.

"Do you think she'll get upset if she sees it in your driveway?" I asked.

"Probably not. She can't see all the driveway from her window and she probably won't recognize it as her old car."

"Okay. I'll sell it to you. I'll get the title and come by tomorrow to settle it and give you the keys."

I was glad I already had mom's power of attorney. I was able to transfer the title and cancel the car insurance. Mom would have some money and one less bill to pay.

The next day I walked to the Debosiers' house before going inside to see my mom. She was waiting for me and when I handed her the title to the car and all sets of keys, she handed me a pouch containing exactly ten thousand dollars in cash. I had never held that much cash in my life. I had Mrs. Debosier walk next door and drive the car back to her house before I went in to visit. It was a short visit and I just said I was coming by to check on her, but that I had to go home soon.

When I got home, I couldn't resist taking the money out of the pouch and holding it. I was going to open a joint checking account with my power of attorney the next day and deposit all of it to be used for my mom's expenses. But just for that night, I got to hold ten thousand dollars in my hands. I spread the bills out like a fan and had my picture taken with all that money. Even though it wasn't mine, it was fun.

I opened the account the next morning under both my name and my mother's; however, I made sure I was the only one authorized to sign on the account. I then got checks and a debit card. Using the power of attorney, I went through the necessary paperwork and red tape to have her Social Security and my dad's army retirement money automatically deposited into the new account every month. While she was still in her house, I knew that moving her would be the next step, and that it would take money.

42

EACH TIME ONE OF the Bees tried to mention moving out of her home, they were met by angry, indignant resistance from my mother.

Peggy is the sweetest of all of us. Her voice is so soft, it's barely above a whisper. She is not confrontational and is always trying to please. While her soothing demeanor elicits calm and comfort from the listener, she is not apt to argue back if the listener disagrees with her.

I can almost hear their conversation now:

"Mother, wouldn't it be nice if you could live someplace smaller? You wouldn't have to climb any stairs. You could have other people clean for you. And you would probably have lots of friends around you. Y'all would have so much fun together."

"No! It wouldn't be fun and I'm not leaving my house!"

"Okay. You don't have to. I was just thinking how much easier it would be for you and I just think you would have fun and be happy."

"No. I would not be happy and I'm not moving."

And that would be the end of the argument.

Katherine is the most practical of the Bees. She carefully examines pros and cons of any situation and tries to make an informed decision based on all of the information available. (Except if she and Cotty are trying to decide where to eat. That's where her decision-making abilities hit a brick wall!)

"Mom, you've already had one broken hip. You cannot continue to live in a house where the only bedroom and full bathroom are upstairs. You should not be climbing stairs and you should be using your walker when you do walk."

"I don't need that walker! I do just fine without it. And I don't have any problems climbing stairs."

"Well, you are at serious risk of falling. You need to be in a place where you live on the ground level with no stairs. And you need to be eating better. You could move to a place that has someone cook your meals for you. It's not practical or safe for you to stay in this house alone."

"I've already told you. Nothing is wrong with me. I do not need to move and that's that! Now just stop."

Another argument lost.

Being the only two in Baton Rouge, Jane and I had already lost the moving argument several times. This was going to be complicated.

We started out by researching facilities in Baton Rouge. There was some money left in my dad's retirement and the money in the joint bank account, but that wouldn't last very long. We would need to sell the house to be able to afford a place with the care my mother required.

Peggy brought home brochures from all over town, everything from assisted living, nursing homes, and special facilities that focused on memory care. But, without forcing her out against her will, we would not be able to move my mom without a fight.

While the doctors felt she needed full nursing care, I don't believe any of us were ready to go that far and we knew that my mom would be absolutely miserable in such a setting. Even though that's what she had always told us to do. She didn't think she was "like that." Nothing was wrong, according to her.

There was one place we thought she might consider. A place near her home called Southside Gardens had individual apartments as well as an assisted living facility. One of the ladies in her bridge group had already moved to an apartment there and had hosted bridge there several times. We figured if she knew someone who already lived there and was assured of having her own place, we might be able to get her to agree to move into an apartment. It wasn't assisted living, but the place included cleaning service, a cafeteria that served meals, and each apartment had a kitchen should one want to cook for themselves. It also included several activities, games, and field trips.

We brought it up to my mom.

"Absolutely not! I told you I'm not leaving this house. Now you can just stop talking about it!"

Now it was time for the Queen Bee and Bee Number 3, Jane. I wasn't about to be kind and practical, and Jane was the queen of getting away with tricks. We met in advance with the director of Southside Gardens, who knew my mom from growing up in her neighborhood. He let us know there was a one bedroom apartment available. That's when we let him in on our plan.

I brought Jane along with me on one of mom's regular doctor visits to have her blood work checked. On the way home, I turned left into Southside Gardens. My mom began hollering.

"What are you doing? Bring me home! I'm not going to live here!"

"Of course you're not going to live here," I replied, "We're just going to visit some of your friends. They haven't seen you in a while and I told them I would bring you over."

"Oh. Well, okay. But just to visit."

We started with a tour of the apartment she had already been in for bridge. Her friend showed her around and talked about how wonderful the place was, how much fun she had been having since she moved there, and how easy her life had become without all that cooking and cleaning to do. Mom's demeanor softened just a little.

Next, we visited the cafeteria and entertainment area. We made sure lunch was just ending so that the room would be full to capacity. And just as if she was back at church or a party twenty years earlier, she was off talking. She seemed to know half of the people in there. She talked and visited with old friends for over an hour. I even saw my old kindergarten teacher, who remembered me from when I was five years old.

After an hour or so of visiting, we ushered her to the car. On the way home, she was smiling.

"You know what? I think I might like living in one of those apartments."

"I wish I could live in one," Jane replied, "I would love to have someone cook meals when I don't feel like it."

I said, "I wish I could move there! I would love someone cleaning my place twice a week. And it has a pool! I would just read by the pool all day and eat the meals they make. It's like a resort. Like you're permanently on vacation."

Jane said, "Okay Virginia, it's a deal. As soon as we can, we're going to move there, too!"

By the time we pulled into the driveway of her house, we not only had her talked into moving to the apartment, we had her excited about it. Walking into her dirty kitchen and realizing she was about to be alone again sealed the deal even further. Her mind was made up.

Jane and I met with the director. He showed us the apartment Mom would be living in. I signed the paperwork and paid the deposit and the first month's rent. Then he told us the places were completely cleaned and redone between guests and that he would need her wallpaper and paint choices as soon as possible, sending us to the store that their painters used.

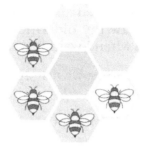

43

NOW THAT MY MOTHER had become the child, and the Bees were the caregivers, it was time to become a team. We were all in this together. It hurt each of us to lose our mother, but we hadn't lost her yet. She was alive. But instead of being the person we went to for advice, comfort, and love, we had to be the ones to make sure she was taken care of, safe, fed, and bathed. As her personality became more childlike, she became the baby we were all responsible for. These Four Bees, with four personalities, would be the team to handle this task. Without one, it would be impossible, but together we could do anything.

Jane and I had the task of picking wallpaper and paint. The director of Southside Gardens had sent us to the representative at the store which handled their account. We were shown samples of wallpaper and paint from an assortment previously approved by the facility.

Almost in unison, we chose, "That, that, and that." We were done and walked away from the shop.

Next, we had to figure out what to move to her apartment and what to do with everything else. The bedroom was much smaller than the master bedroom at her house, so we chose to bring the queen-sized bed that had been in Katherine's old room rather than the king that was my mom and dad's. We knew she would want the blue La-Z-Boy recliner, even though by this time it was starting to have the same odor as her car. We chose a sofa from the formal living room because the couches in the family room were nine feet long and would never fit into an apartment. We picked a dresser, end tables, dining set, and a coffee table.

Then we began to choose decorations. We made sure she had several pictures of family all over the apartment, framed on the walls, dresser and tables, and even held with magnets on the refrigerator. We also chose art from her walls at home. We brought the Williamsburg print we had given our parents for their 50th wedding anniversary. She loved birds and had several framed Audubon prints of different species throughout her home, as well as porcelain music boxes in shapes of her favorite species. We chose what could fit without making it too crowded or cluttered, but enough to make it seem like home.

When moving day arrived after Christmas, we took turns distracting my mom while things were moved from her house to the apartment. We spent all day arranging the furniture, hanging the pictures, making the bed with linens from her house, and putting away her clothes and toiletries. We did not want her to feel as if she was in a strange place. It was a long and exhausting day, but finally, we were ready to bring her over.

She did not seem hesitant as we drove her to the place. When she went in and saw all of her things, she actually seemed happy to be there. It was as if she had been secretly wanting to get away from all the clutter of her house and live in a smaller place, but if she did it on her own, it would somehow be admitting that something was wrong with her, or that she couldn't handle her house on her own, and she was not ready to admit any such thing.

We showed her around the place and where everything had been put away. Then she settled into her blue chair and turned on the television. I know it was much harder on us to leave her there that first night than it was on her. We all knew she needed to move out of her house, but actually moving her meant the end of an era. No more meals at her kitchen table, no more Sunday School class Christmas parties, and no more going home to Mom. I bent to give her a kiss and watched her as I closed the door behind me, thinking of her all alone in a new place for the first time in over half a century.

I held everything in until I got home and then began sobbing. I just flopped down on the bed and let the tears flow. She was alive, but everything was different. I was just crying out, "I want my mom!" But what I wanted was no longer there. Things had forever changed and there was no going back. I let the tears flow until I couldn't cry anymore.

That night, Katherine came over to eat at my house. She was sleeping at my mom's house—now my mom's old house. But we had decided to grill steaks and celebrate finally finishing the move. I had never been a martini person, but had recently discovered how to make a Cosmopolitan, or "the chick martini." I felt sophisticated. Katherine and I continued making them and drinking them as the food was being prepared.

I don't know if it was because I was drinking on an empty stomach, or if all of the tears from earlier had dehydrated my body, or if my body just revolted from being fed so much hard liquor, but before the dinner was even ready, I was on the floor vomiting in the half-bath off of my kitchen. And once I started, I could not stop. While everyone tried to eat their steaks and ignore the awful retching sounds coming from the other side of the door, I dry-heaved and threw up for hours. Finally, when my body felt all the evil of the day was out of it, I was able to move to my bed and sleep.

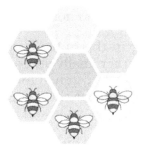

44

THE MOVE TOOK LONGER to accomplish than the doctors had wanted, and it was not a full nursing care facility, but it was a step, and one we were able to convince our mom to go along with voluntarily. She settled in nicely to apartment living. She attended meals in the cafeteria and appreciated the cleaning service that came twice a week.

I kept up the routine of taking her to get her hair done every Thursday morning, with my dog in the back seat. She still smiled every time she turned around and looked at that huge grin on my Golden Retriever. She remained extremely stubborn about using her walker, so I would escort her up to the door of Pace's when I dropped her off. I would then go home, shower, get dressed for work, and one of the hairdressers would walk her out to my car where I was waiting for her when she was done.

Jane and I continued to take her to doctor appointments and to the grocery store. We took turns visiting her and stocking her pantry with snacks she enjoyed that didn't require much in the way of preparation. We sent out announcement cards to all the friends and family in her address book notifying them of her new address so she would continue to receive mail and calls from her friends.

If Katherine or Peggy was in town, they would take her to appointments and help as much as possible. On one particular visit, Peggy and I went together with my mom to her family doctor for a checkup. I figured she was just having bloodwork to adjust her Coumadin levels and not much else. Boy was I wrong.

After hours of waiting in the outer waiting room and in the examining room, Dr. Parker finally entered. He talked with us as he checked Mom's vitals and listened to her heart. Next, he had her disrobe and cover herself with a sheet. Then he proceeded to scoot her to the edge of the table and pull out stirrups.

"What!?" I thought to myself, "This is not the gynecologist office!" I didn't even know they had stirrups in the family doctor room.

As Peggy and I took turns looking at each other in horror and staring at the ground in complete embarrassment, he proceeded to give my mother a complete pelvic exam and pap smear, acting nonchalantly as he continued to make casual conversation with us. I was hoping my mom's dementia was bad enough that she did not realize what was happening, because I know the old Mildred Evans would have been outraged by this. I think Peggy and I were scarred for life after witnessing that doctor visit.

Not to be outdone when we came home to tell the other Bees about it, Jane related what had happened to her the last time she had to take Mom to the doctor.

"They made me go to the bathroom with her to get a urine sample!" she started, "And Mom didn't know what to do, so I had to hold the cup between her legs so she could pee in it. It was awful. I can't unsee that view. It is going to be seared in my brain and haunt me forever!"

Never did we know that we would be first-hand witnesses to my mother's gross loss of privacy as well as her memory. While we had to laugh to get through it, it was so incredibly sad as well.

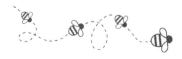

Not every doctor visit was that terrifying. On one of our follow-up visits to the neurologist, the doctor was simply checking to see if she had gotten any worse or if the disease had slowed its progression. It was difficult to tell if anything had changed, so we decided to keep her on the Aricept, despite its $350 per month price tag. And we agreed she needed to stay on the Zoloft to help with depression and irritability.

On our way out of the building, I noticed a lady unloading boxes from the trunk of her car onto a small dolly. It turned out she was a pharmaceutical rep making her rounds to the neurology department.

"Look, Mom," I said, as I stared down at the boxes, "She sells the exact medicine you take."

The lady overheard me and looked up, "Really, she takes Aricept and Zoloft?"

I showed her the prescriptions in my hand and explained that we had just come from the neurologist.

She asked where my car was and followed me over to it. When I opened the back, she stacked the boxes of samples of both medicines into my car. I thanked her over and over, realizing that she probably just saved us over $1,000. She said she was happy to help and returned to her car to load more samples onto her dolly and go about her rounds.

I wish I knew who she was to thank her again. It's such a blessing to come across such random acts of kindness, especially when dealing with such a dreadful circumstance.

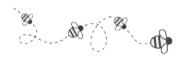

Besides the hair and doctor appointments, my mom had a few other activities. Her friends from bridge continued to pick her up and take her to play on Thursdays, and Dot Howell would occasionally take her to the alumni center to serve as a docent.

Dot Debosier would drive her to visit my Uncle Charlie and take her on bus trips to the casino.

While she had some activities to keep her busy, whenever I visited I would find her sitting in the blue chair. She sat quietly, not reading, not watching TV—just sitting. I would wonder what thoughts went through her head. She was more and more forgetful. She had trouble completing sentences and thoughts. But she seemed content with the apartment and her routine.

It was around this time that Bill called me at my office. I had not heard from him since the fight in the hospital when my mom had her aorta surgery. I was completely caught off guard.

"Well, hello Virginia, this is Bill,"

"Hi. How are you?" I was confused, hesitant.

"I'm very well, thank you. I am living in Boulder, Colorado now. It's wonderful. We get to ski in the winter. The mountains are beautiful. We are doing extremely well."

"That's good."

"Also, I now collect rare birds as a hobby. I have a basement in our home in Colorado. We have covered the floor and walls in vinyl that can be washed down. We keep several rare bird species in there. I'm actually in Lafayette now to pick up a new bird for my collection. I figured since I'm so close I might go visit Mother," he and Peggy always referred to her as "mother" while the rest of us just called her "Mom."

"Okay. Do you need the address?"

"No, I was just letting you know that I would be in town shortly and would be visiting her."

"Alright, well, thanks for calling."

"Okay. Goodbye." And he hung up. As usual, he didn't ask me how I—or anyone else—was. But I was used to this by now and wanted to get off the phone as soon as possible.

I hung up the phone and called the Bees.

He was going to visit "Mother." The locks were still on the house and she didn't have too many things in the apartment, so there was no worry about him taking anything. Maybe it was a good thing. She would probably be happy to have a visit from her son.

Late that afternoon, he called me again.

"Hello Virginia. This is Bill."

"Hi."

"Mother would like to go to an awards banquet at the LSU alumni center tonight. Would it be okay with you if I took her?" I guess she had continued to get her mail and invitations for alumni events.

"It's fine with me, if you want to. You need to make sure she is appropriately dressed for it."

"Oh, she's already decided on her dress and has it on. She looks fine."

"Well, as long as you're okay bringing her, I don't see any reason not to. Have a good time."

"Oh, we will. Thank you for letting me take her."

I guess part of me appreciated that he asked. The last time we had seen each other was when he was fighting to be the boss of Mom in the hospital after having been absent for years. Now, he was deferring to me. Was he acknowledging the work we had done to get her to this point? Were we appreciated? I don't know. He didn't say. But it did mean something that he asked. Maybe he had changed. Maybe he wasn't selfish anymore. It was time to give him a break.

My new attitude changed when Jane called me after 11 p.m.

"You are not even going to believe what just happened!" she started.

"What?"

"The secretary of the director of the alumni center just called me to ask me for Mom's address."

"Why?"

"It seems Bill did not go with Mom to the banquet tonight. He just dropped her off there and left. When it was over, everyone left and Mom was just wandering around alone and confused. The lady offered to drive her home, but Mom didn't know where she lived. She called me to get Mom's address so she could take her home. He just left her there alone and she was the last person there."

"You have got to be kidding me!"

"No! I'm serious. They said she sat at the banquet alone and no one picked her up!"

"I swear, when he was on the phone with me I totally assumed he was going with her. He asked if he could take her to the banquet. I didn't think for a minute that he meant he would just be dropping her off. Did he just assume one of us would pick her up? I never saw the invitation. I wouldn't even have known what time to pick her up."

"I know! I'm so embarrassed," Jane said, "Now everyone at the alumni center probably thinks we don't even care about our own mother!"

I was in shock. I was not expecting this at all. It was just the beginning of embarrassments this whole situation would cause, but this one was caused by Bill, not by Mom. How could he do this?! Did he not think of anybody except himself?!

Ding! Ding! Ding! We have a winner!

"Of course he hasn't changed. I should have expected this. I should have seen it coming."

"There's no way you could have known," said Jane, "He acted like he was going to take her. It's only natural to think that meant he would stay there with her and bring her back."

"He has absolutely no clue about her condition. How could he not have noticed how much she has changed?! How she could not be left alone in a public place?!"

We would have to be very careful about who took Mom anywhere and what they would be doing to take care of her and get her home safely. While I was still embarrassed, I was so grateful to the kind lady who stayed around waiting for my mother to get a ride and then bringing her home once she realized no one was coming for her.

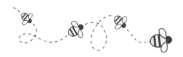

Shortly after this incident, Dot Howell called and asked me if she could take Mom to another event at the alumni center. I told her that I appreciated her offer, but that I didn't think it was a good idea. She said she had already talked to my mom about it and that she wanted to go and was excited about it. It would be a shame not to let her. I explained about what happened the last time Mom attended one of these events.

"Oh no! This is different. She will be next to me the entire time and I will be driving her back to her apartment right when it is over."

"Well, in that case, I guess it will be okay."

When it came time for her to pick up my mom for the dinner, I received another call from Dot Howell, only this time she was aggravated.

"I'm over here to get your mother, and she is not even ready to go. She is sitting in that chair in a nightgown tucked into some sweatpants and acting like she's just going to wear that!"

"I understand. I've tried to explain. She's not the same. She doesn't need to be going out in public."

"Well, she could go out in public if you would come over here and make sure she is properly dressed."

"When you called and asked if you could take her, I didn't know that meant I needed to go get her dressed. I'm sorry."

"Never mind. I'll find something for her to change into and see if I can get her to wear it. But we need to hurry, we're already running late."

"Okay. Good Luck. Thank you." And the call was over.

The last time a friend took my mother to the alumni center, I received a call at work. This time, she had fallen on her way in. While she hadn't broken any bones this time, her dentures had pierced through her bottom lip. Because she was taking blood thinners, the hole in her lip was bleeding profusely. An ambulance had taken her to the emergency room.

Jane and I made it to the hospital once again to sit with her. By the time I arrived, her lip had been stitched up, but she was confused and kept picking at the stitches with her hands. We waited all day to speak to a doctor while my mother moaned in pain. A nurse walked in and asked her what medications she was taking.

"I don't take any medicine," my mother said.

"She takes Aricept, Zoloft, and Coumadin." I told the nurse.

"I'm sorry ma'am, but I need her to answer the question, not you." She was being rude now.

"Do you need her to answer? Or do you need to know what medications she takes? Those are going to be completely different answers."

"Well, I guess you can tell me, then."

I told her the medications once more and asked when a doctor would see her and when she could get something for pain. She replied that she could not have anything for her pain until after the doctor determined if she had any further injuries to her head. Meanwhile, my mom was moaning.

Late that afternoon, they moved her from the emergency room to a regular room, yet she still had not been seen by a doctor and was still moaning. After a few hours of this, I completely lost it. I stormed down to the nurses' station.

"My mother fell at 8 this morning. She has stitches from a gaping hole in her bottom lip. She is moaning in pain. And no doctor has seen her all day."

"Well, a physician's assistant saw her earlier today."

"But they didn't give her anything for pain, order any tests, or do anything but move her to a room! If someone doesn't give her something in the next ten minutes, I'm going to the Walgreens across the street to buy her some fucking Tylenol!"

I was at my limit. Nice face gone. I had been ignored by everyone at this hospital since early morning. Jane convinced me to leave. A doctor did come check her, gave her some pain medicine, and she was discharged early the following morning. I made a decision that she was not going to the LSU alumni center again. Ever!

I believe it was more difficult for my mom's friends to accept the changes in her than it was for us. She had always been the strong one. The dominant friend. The driver on all the road trips. The loud one who talked to everyone in the room. To see her in her new state was particularly sad, maybe because they were closer to her age. Would this happen to them one day? I think mostly they just missed their friend. It was probably easier if they could blame her condition on how we were handling her care rather than accept that the old Mildred was gone.

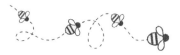

As much as I was against anyone taking my mom out in public, we continued to pick her up and bring her home for holidays. The idea of her sitting alone on Thanksgiving or Christmas was unbearable, so we would go get her, or send Katherine if she was in town, and take her to either my house or Jane's, whichever one of us was hosting the meal.

One Thanksgiving at my house when it was storming outside, Katherine carefully helped her out of the rain and into my house. Once inside, she began looking at all the food. We made sure not to pick her up too early, as we didn't want her away from her place for too long.

Then she started going down the row of dishes I was setting out so that everyone could begin to fix their plates. She reached her hand into the pot of green beans, took some out, and shoved them in her mouth. *Ugh!* We were disgusted. The old Mildred would have been so appalled at herself. We just let it go and began to have our dinner. I'm not sure any of us ate the green beans that day.

The following Christmas, the dinner was at Jane's house. We had all of her family and ours, including my cousin Cecil, his son Patrick, and Patrick's girlfriend at the time, Jenn. She was so cute and sweet and we all adored her. This was her first Christmas to be away from her home to eat with Patrick's family and we wanted her to feel welcome.

Katherine picked up Mom and made sure she was appropriately dressed before bringing her over to Jane's. She ushered her through the kitchen to the table, making sure she kept her hands out of the food. Katherine fixed her a plate and a glass of iced tea and placed it in front of her. When everyone had their food and the blessing was said, we began eating Christmas dinner. The food was amazing, just like Mom's used to be. The conversation was pleasant. Everything was going fine.

Until Katherine took Mom's plate to the kitchen in order to bring her a dessert. That's when my mom decided to remove her dentures from her mouth, pick them clean with the tines of her fork, and drop them into her iced tea to soak for a while!

We looked at each other in horror. We had a stranger at the table. She wasn't family. And THIS was going to be the story she had to remember about Christmas with the Evans sisters! I wanted to throw up my dinner. No way could I eat dessert with those teeth staring at me from the light brown liquid in the glass next to me.

We decided then and there that we could visit Mom on holidays. We could bring her a plate of food and presents to unwrap. But under no circumstances were we checking her out and taking her in public ever again.

I know she would have wanted it that way. I think she probably tries to haunt me to this day for letting her out in public all those times before this incident. Mildred Evans, the high-fashion-hair-done social butterfly, picking her dentures and dropping them in her tea!

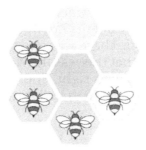

45

LESS THAN ONE YEAR after we moved mom into her apartment, we began to receive complaints from the staff at Southside Gardens. The cleaning staff complained of the horrible stench of urine in her apartment and the constantly soiled sheets on her bed. The director was concerned because she was no longer coming to meals in the cafeteria. And it was becoming apparent to Jane and me that she was not taking her medicine as directed. Once again, a move needed to be made.

After researching the different facilities and costs, and considering my mom's resistance to change, the Bees decided to move her to the assisted living facility in Southside Gardens. This way, she would only be moving across the parking lot and not to a completely new area.

We toured the assisted living facility without my mom first. Her room would have a twin bed and room for her chair. It had built in drawers for her clothes and she would have her own bathroom with safety rails. Her caretakers would assist her with bathing and getting to and from her meals and activities. Since it was not a nursing facility, however, they would not be allowed to give medicine to her. This was a downside, but we thought if we put the pills in a container labeled with the days of the week, maybe she would take them each day.

They brought us downstairs to the cafeteria and activity room. It resembled the one at the apartment complex except for having more employees, more residents in wheelchairs, and less activity and discussion going on. There was one perk that had my mind made up immediately that this was the right place for my mom. It had a beauty parlor! That's right. She could get her hair done right in the building. No more early Thursday drives to Pace's! I was sold.

Rather than just start moving my mom's things from her apartment, Jane and I decided it was time for a fresh start. First, we went to the local Sam's Club and purchased a vinyl recliner chair for her new room. The old blue one had soaked up too much urine and was probably the main source of the awful stench. We then purchased a twin sized "Bed In A Bag" set that contained a comforter and matching sheets for the twin bed in her new room.

Next, we filled the top drawer with adult pull-ups. It was time to finally make my mom wear diapers. If she was resistant to using her walker, she was downright defiant about wearing any kind of adult incontinence products, but it was not going to be her choice anymore. It had gotten progressively worse and she could no longer go on soiling herself and her furnishings. We decided against moving any of her underwear to the new room so that her only choice would be to wear the pullups.

We got the bed and chair set up, then moved as many of the pictures that would fit into the new room. Then we walked my mom across the parking lot and up the elevator to show her the space. To our surprise, she smiled with the joy of a small child. She touched the new bedding and ran her fingers over the new recliner.

"This is mine?" she asked.

"Yes indeed. It's all yours. What do you think?"

"Oh, it's nice. I like this bed. I like this room."

We were able to leave her in her newly decorated and clean room feeling much better than we felt after the first move. Now it was time to clean out the apartment.

The blue recliner chair went to the dumpster. There's not a thrift store or garage sale that I would have forced that chair on. The smell would have immediately taken over any room, and no one should be subjected to that. Her underwear went into the dumpster as well. Anything of value that someone might want to keep for sentimental reasons was taken to her old house and everything else was thrown away.

For several weeks, I begged and pleaded with my mom to use the beauty parlor in her building. At first she flat refused, insisting I take her to Pace's. I tried a few Thursdays of being "sick" or "having a meeting at work" leaving her hair to go flat and dirty. Eventually, she gave in to one of the caregiver's offers to take her and, after her first visit to the in-house beauty parlor, she was fine with it. And I was done with my Thursday morning errand for good.

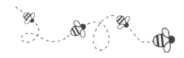

With this move, the cost of my mom's care was growing. It was time to sell her house. Jane had just earned her real estate agent's license, so this would become her first listing. It couldn't be sold until all the stuff was out. This was going to be a feat of massive proportion.

Since my father's death, the house had become so disorganized. In what was once his drawing room were stacks and boxes of papers. Some contained old L.L.Bean catalogs from the 1980s and back issues of *Southern Living*. But sometimes, tucked in between such "junk" would be something important, like my birth certificate, or one of the war letters. This required us to go through every piece of paper in the house and try to separate them into garbage as well as stacks for each sibling and then a general stack that we would keep, but didn't know who would be doing the keeping.

Every room was filled with furniture. Every kitchen cabinet was full. Two kitchen drawers were filled to the top with a variety of plastic lids which had no matching containers to be found. There were so many closets to go through. My dad, the architect, did not waste any space; therefore, there was storage abound, and each nook and cranny was filled with a half a century worth of stuff.

I started with what had been my bedroom. It had not changed since I was in college. There were bulletin boards on the walls which held photos and corsages from dances in high school and college, and boxes of letters my friends and family had written to me at camp or at school over the years. The two closets were filled with clothes from the 1980s and 1990s that hadn't been touched for years. Just looking at all the dresses made memories flash through my head like a movie. I could remember each dance I went to in each dress and who my date was. I remembered shopping with my mom in Dallas and in Baton Rouge for the perfect outfit for every event. Wow, it had been fun to shop with her. I missed everything and just wanted to go back in time.

Since I couldn't go backwards, I began going through everything. I started by taking all of my nice dresses and clothes to goodwill. I narrowed down all my knick knacks to one small Rubbermaid box and forced myself to move everything else downstairs to the trash or garage sale piles. I removed all the pictures from the bulletin boards and placed them in another Rubbermaid box with the thousands of photos already stuffed into boxes at my house.

When I began pulling boxes out from under my old bed, I discovered once again how much of a recycler my dad was. I pulled out two boxes completely filled with what seemed like hundreds of the small, black, plastic, cylindrical containers that used to hold 35mm film way before anyone had a digital camera. I knew he took a lot of pictures for work and would take some at home when he had to finish up a roll and have it developed in time for a court appearance or deposition, but I had no idea that he had kept every single plastic container. I suppose he thought one day he would find a use for them, just as he had for the baby food jars holding the hardware in his workshop.

Having my room cleared out was only a small step in the process of selling the house. The living room had become a depository for what would be put in a garage sale. The couches in the family room held everything that we felt someone would want to keep. I'm not sure who came up with the idea to work from the top down, but it seemed like a good strategy.

I was out of town for Thanksgiving when Peggy, Tim, Aaron, Charlotte, and Katherine came into town and cleared out the attic. The new part of the house had a walk-up attic where one could fully stand up with the area of nearly the entire square footage of the house's footprint. Like every closet or cabinet, it was full. They worked tirelessly, carrying everything down the two flights of stairs to the first floor, then again going through the separation process.

Junky old toys and stuffed animals were in bags next to chests of World War II artifacts and family heirlooms that would be valuable to someone. Everything had to be sorted before anything could be thrown out. That time they all cleaned the attic was the first Thanksgiving I ever spent away from family, and I have to say I was thankful not to be at home that weekend.

After the massive garage sale, which did not bring in nearly enough money to compensate for the effort that went into it, it was time to divide up everything else. Peggy, the sweetest but still a Bee, was the only one of us who ever kept in touch with Bill. When it came time to contact him about any family business, she got tagged for the task.

She let him know that we were going to be dividing up things from the house. We had already decided to draw numbers and take turns in numerical order picking something we wished to keep. He told her he didn't want anything, which was a surprise considering all the things he tried to take after my dad died. But Peggy, wanting everything to be fair, drew a number for him and chose things she thought he might like to ship to him later.

Once we had all made our choices and taken everything else to be donated or thrown away, we were down to approximately five Rubbermaid boxes of things and papers that no one wanted to claim, but no one wanted to discard. On the morning of the closing, I went to visit my childhood home for the last time. I said goodbye to my old room with tears in my eyes. Then I walked through my parents' room, Dad's drawing room, the kitchen that had produced countless heavenly, mouth-watering meals, and the family room that had held the twenty-foot-tall Christmas trees and all the parties that went along with that season. As I walked out of the front door for the last time and locked it behind me, I packed up the remaining boxes of stuff no one wanted and loaded them into my car.

After the sale of the house, I took the money from my parents' home to an investment friend of mine. I described the situation, that my mom was in assisted living, that she would need more and more care, and that her Social Security, my dad's army retirement money, and the proceeds from this house would have to pay for it. He understood and explained he would do his best to make it last as long as possible while transferring a monthly amount to her checking account to help cover the expenses of her care. The cost of the assisted living was not too much more than the apartment, so this seemed reasonable. But the costs were about to go up again.

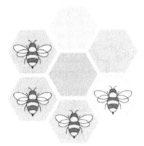

46

WHILE MOVING EVERYTHING OUT of her house to get it ready to sell, I had been keeping my eye out for Mom's safe deposit box key. I remembered her showing it to me the night before she went into the hospital for the aneurysm on her aorta. Once her house got in such disarray, the key was impossible to find. There were at least a hundred keys in different drawers and cabinets, but it was impossible to identify the correct one for the safe deposit box.

Jane and I started making it our mission to find out what was in this box. After all, mom had been cashing all those checks from those credit card companies and had nothing to show for it, so maybe she was stashing it in the box. Also, both of my parents lived through the Great Depression. Maybe they didn't believe in stock market investing and had stashed decades worth of cash savings in the box. Or maybe there was some jewelry we didn't know about.

I contacted the bank. Without the key, we would need to pay a $400 fee to have the box drilled open. Also, they would need to see my power of attorney as well as my father's succession documents. Well, that was easy. I showed up with all of the paperwork, ready to write a check and open the box.

"We will also need your father's death certificate."

Well, this was getting more complicated. Among the clutter in the house, none of us had come across my father's death certificate. "That's okay," I thought, "I'll just call the Office of Vital Records."

In Louisiana, the Office of Vital Records, a division of the Department of Health and Human Services, is located in New Orleans rather than Baton Rouge. After Hurricane Katrina, they ran this office at less than a snail's pace.

I was told to mail a request in writing along with a check for $7.00 and they would send the certificate. Despite several calls to their office, we received no response...until it had been more than six months. At that point, I received a letter from them that my check for $7.00 was more than 180 days old, so I would have to send a new request with a new check to get the certificate!

So, it takes MORE THAN 180 days to process the request for a death certificate, but the check to pay for the death certificate expires in 180 days! Who's on First!?

By now I was going crazy at our state's ridiculous failure to provide services and its crazy red tape. I sent the new request and a new check, along with letters to the Director of Health and Human Services, the Governor, and any other official I could think of who might help.

Within a few weeks, the death certificate finally came. I brought it to the lady in charge of the safe deposit boxes at the bank, paid the fee for the drilling, and she set up an appointment for us to come back and examine the box when the security company would be there to drill it open.

That morning, Jane and I could not control our excitement as we drove downtown to find out what was in the box. We let our imaginations run wild with what magnificent riches we were about to discover. Jane even took a detour past her dream house which happened to be for sale, just in case we were all about to become millionaires.

We entered the bank and were escorted to the vault where the safe deposit boxes were kept. The man from the security company carried a ladder as well as his drilling equipment. We watched as he climbed towards a box at the very top.

"That box looks a little small." I whispered to Jane.

"I know. I was hoping it would be one of those big ones at the bottom."

"Oh well, it could still be full of cash."

We waited impatiently as he drilled through the keyhole. Finally he removed the box from its slot and began his descent down the ladder.

"It looks really light." Jane said.

"I know. And it was quiet when he turned it. I didn't hear anything slide around in there."

With great anticipation, we opened the lid to the box. And what was inside?

A COPY of my mother's will! That's it! Nothing else! I already had the original of this will. I didn't need to go through a year of red tape, headaches, and money to get a copy of it. I think the lady at the bank was secretly satisfied.

Jane and I drove home feeling more defeated than I can remember. No jewelry. No cash. Nothing. Why did we even try? Oh well, another story to laugh about. I always told people about the moment the man pulled out the box and tipped it sideways.

"I just knew I would hear a giant thud as the Blue Heart Jewel from *Titanic* slid to the other side of the box," I would tell them, "But no. Nothing. Just a copy of an old will and a box full of disappointment."

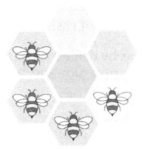

47

Jane called me one morning in a fit. I immediately asked what was wrong.

"Those workers at Southside Gardens called me in the middle of the night because apparently Mom pooed all over her bed and poo was everywhere in her room! They needed me to come get her sheets and wash them and return them! It was so disgusting! Poo was everywhere! I took the whole comforter and sheet set and threw them in the dumpster. The workers objected, saying that was good bedding, but I wasn't about to put that mess in my car. We need to go buy a new comforter set. Now!"

"Are you kidding me? I knew mom peed herself all the time, but poo?"

"Yes, and it was everywhere! And they don't handle that at assisted living. So they called ME in the middle of the night!"

"Shit!" I knew this was much worse than buying a new comforter. It was bad if she was in a place that wouldn't make her take her medicine, but if the employees wouldn't clean her poo sheets in the middle of the night, it was time for another level of care.

We purchased the new "Bed In A Bag" set and made up the bed in my mom's room then called the out-of-town Bees. It was time to move again. This was becoming exhausting.

Jane and I began to visit several different facilities all over town. One thing that stood out to me about nursing homes (and child care centers, too, as I now know) is the smell. It's a combination of cleaning solution and urine. It's as if, no matter how many employees they hire, there is no way to have every resident dry and the entire place clean at the same time. As soon as they've changed the last diaper, the first person is wet again. So the smell is a constant.

Now we were looking at nursing homes. "When I get like that, lock me up in a nursing home and forget about me." The words kept running through our minds as we toured each place. As long as we could call it an apartment or assisted living, it didn't feel so bad. But these places were bad. Not that they weren't nice facilities. They all had lovely grounds, kind staff, good food, and a high level of care, but they were sad. I could tell this was the last place these people would live before they died. I didn't want to ever live in one.

Jane and I made a pact with each other. *When we get "like that," we're moving to Oregon where assisted suicide is legal and we're just going to end it!* Decision made, that's final. But we both knew that when or if we get "like that," we won't be going to Oregon or anywhere else, because we will adamantly declare to everyone that we're NOT "like that." That's the whole problem with Alzheimer's. You can't plan how you're going to handle the disease, because once you have it, you don't remember any plans. Your loved ones have to make the decisions and make sure you are taken care of and you live in a dream world where nothing is wrong with you.

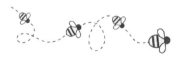

After looking all over town and comparing our options, we decided on a facility called Cypress Manor. The grounds on this one were beautiful. It was set back far from the road and surrounded by ancient oaks and acres of lovely landscaping. Also, and what mainly factored into our decision, it had a sister facility, where, should my mom run out of money, she could move free of charge once her resources were exhausted.

While signing up to move my mom in, we decided to pay the higher price for her to have her own room rather than share one with a roommate. That just made it seem even more like a hospital and we weren't ready for that. They asked if we would be using their adult diapers or supplying our own. I asked the cost and they told me it would be $4.00 per diaper. No, we'd be supplying her diapers. Not only did Cypress Manor have a beauty parlor where Mom could get her hair done, it had a doctor and nurses. I wouldn't have to drive her to any more doctor appointments! She would be seen by their doctor and her medications would be monitored, prescribed, and administered by the staff. It seemed like with each move, we would have less work to do. But also with each move, we lost a part of my mom we would never get back.

I know Peggy had doubts about our choice; I'm not sure about Katherine. But we did what we thought was best, carefully considering the level of care our mother needed, and the resources she had available to pay for her care. Unfortunately, none of Mildred and Red's children had grown up to be extremely wealthy, or even a little wealthy. None of us could have afforded a home nurse or a nursing home bill. So she would have to live on the money she had left and, as of now, I was in charge of managing it.

Each time she would come into town, Peggy would drive around Baton Rouge and tour other places. She would bring brochures to me from places like St. James and Sunrise among other facilities. I would take the brochures and later set them aside, unread. I had already looked everywhere, compared everything, and the decision had been made.

Once I even offered to give my power of attorney and the checkbook to Peggy if she would take Mom back to Dallas with her.

"Oh no. I couldn't do that. I just thought Mother might be happier in one of these places."

Then Jane and I would beg Katherine to take her to Virginia and put her in a new nursing home which had been built near the mountains and close to Katherine's house. Katherine was much more blunt.

"No way! Y'all are doing a great job. I'll help whenever I'm in town, but y'all are in charge!"

So, Mom lived at Cypress Manor.

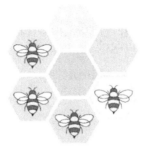

48

ONE OF THE FIRST problems we got a call about was that she had lost her teeth!

"What?"

"She must have left them on her lunch tray. I don't think they're comfortable for her. She's always taking them out," the nurse told me.

While they had a doctor on site, it was up to me to take her to the dentist. I took her back to the same young man who had been schmoozing her out of her football tickets (by now I had changed them into my name and my address and I paid the bill). He took another set of impressions, and several thousand dollars later, I brought my mom back for the final fitting of her new set of dentures.

Another time, I got a complaint call from the staff because my mom had taken all of the clothes out of her drawers and closet and had piled them on the floor. When asked about it, she simply replied that her brother, Charlie, was on his way to pick her up and take her to live with her mama, and he would be there any minute, so she had to pack.

While my Uncle Charlie was still living, he was by no means driving to Baton Rouge, and my grandmother had been dead for eighteen years. Nevertheless, the staff needed someone from the family to calm her down and put away her clothes.

At this point, I was about seven months pregnant with my first child. I could barely bend over with the watermelon-sized belly I was carrying around. Jane and I went to her room together. I would be in charge of talking to her and distracting her while Jane put her clothes away.

As Jane began folding and hanging clothing items from the floor, my mom was frantically complaining.

"Stop that! Leave that there. I'm getting picked up and moving to Mama's and I need to take those things with me!"

Jane gave me a look.

I sat on the bed and looked at my mom, who was sitting in the vinyl recliner.

"It sure has been hot this summer. Have you been going outside much?"

"No. What is she doing?"

"Oh, she's just helping tidy up. You have such a great view from your window. I see a birdfeeder right out there. Do you see many birds?"

"Oh, I don't look out there. I don't see anything. And I'm leaving anyway."

"Now Mom. You aren't going anywhere. Don't you like it here? They take such good care of you. And you not only get your hair done, I see they did your fingernails too. That's such a pretty color."

"Well, I did like that."

"You know what else you'll like?" I kept trying to distract her so Jane could finish putting the clothes away.

"What?" She asked, not expecting to like anything I had to say.

"I'm going to have a baby!" I was so excited to tell her my news. "You're going to have a new granddaughter! Won't that be great?"

Without missing a beat, in the ugliest tone I had ever heard from her she exclaimed, "So! Who's the father?"

Seriously? I was already huge, hormonal, and emotional. All my friends had moms who attended their baby showers, went to the hospital with them, and then helped take care of the baby so the mom could rest. Most of their moms had their own set of carseat, stroller, crib, etc. so they could care for their grandchild at a moment's notice. And this was the slap in the face reaction I got from my own mother.

I looked at Jane, who was horrified, "That's it! I'm out of here! You're on your own!" I said as I stormed out and waited in the car while Jane hurriedly finished putting away the clothes.

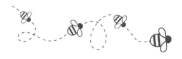

By this time, we no longer had to drive my mom to hair appointments or doctor visits. Jane no longer had to refill her pill organizer once a week. We could visit when we wanted to without the work. But we still got the calls. If I saw Cypress Manor on the caller ID, I would cringe and think, "What now?" Aside from losing her teeth and the clothing incident, most calls were to inform me that she was running low on diapers. I would go to Sam's, get a few of the largest boxes available, and drop them off with her name written with a Sharpie all over the box. (I'm still convinced they used some of hers for other people, but I'm over it.)

Her friends would seldom visit her at Cypress Manor. I remember once Dot Debosier checked her out and drove her to LaRose to see my uncle Charlie. Upon her return to Baton Rouge, she called Jane and asked if she could take Mom back to Cypress Manor for her.

"I have her here at my house and I just can't bear the thought of making her go back to that place! It's just awful. Can you just come get her and take her back there for me?"

Jane agreed, but we still couldn't understand why her friends were reluctant to visit. Dot Howell visited with me once on my mom's birthday. She brought a cake, which we cut in the dining area after singing "Happy Birthday." My mother seemed to enjoy it, but I'm not sure she recognized us or even understood that it was her birthday that we were celebrating.

Sometimes we would visit and bring her a stuffed animal or a doll. She would be thrilled. She was becoming more and more childlike. She would talk about her mama in the present tense as if she was alive. She would talk lovingly about her mama, like she must have felt before her daddy was killed. In her mind, she was younger than thirteen.

There were also times when she would talk as if she were older, maybe college. There was one time when Katherine went to visit. As Katherine entered her room, Mom immediately began questioning her.

"Where's Red? I hope he's not talking to that other woman!" she said, implying he and the other woman were going to be in some serious trouble. I don't believe my father ever stepped out on his wife, so this must have been some distorted college memory. Or just something made up in her head. No one knew what was going on in her brain. Katherine ignored the comment rather than trying to remind her that the love of her life was dead.

After my daughter was born, I would bring her with me to visit my mom. This absolutely delighted her. No more wondering about who the father was. I would make sure Mom was settled into her recliner, then gently hand over her new granddaughter, making sure her head was supported by my mother's arm. My mom could not stop smiling at her! She looked at her with so much love. I think, even if she didn't recognize it, something in her knew this was a special baby, a part of her, and you could feel the joy in the room.

One time Aaron was in town and went to visit Mom at Cypress Manor. He called ahead and asked the caregivers if it would be okay for him to play music in the activity room for the residents on his guitar. They always welcomed free entertainment and frequently hosted children's choirs and school orchestras to play for the patients, so they immediately agreed. Imagine their surprise when he showed up with his electric guitar, amp, and speaker and began giving his own private Metallica cover concert to the room of elderly nursing home patients! They seemed to enjoy the company and the music, even if it wasn't quite their style.

The next time I saw Cypress Manor on the caller ID it was to let me know that my mother had once again lost her dentures! This time I was done. She never liked them. She took them out at the table. She even took them out to eat. I had seen her gum an entire hamburger with those teeth sitting right on the table in front of her. I was through driving her back and forth to the dentist and paying thousands of dollars for something she didn't want anyway. If she wasn't going to wear them, then why bother? Now other siblings probably had different opinions on this decision of mine, but I wasn't going to be the one to put her through that again. It was obvious she hated them, so I just let her go without teeth. To this day, I have pictures of her holding my baby, grinning ear to ear, with that wide open toothless smile. But in her eyes you can see joy.

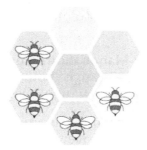

49

THINGS WITH MY MOM had been going well for a while. Katherine and Peggy would come into town. They would go buy some diapers to deliver to Cypress Manor and they would visit with our mom. Then we would have more time to enjoy one another. With her in the nursing home, she was less work. Once the diapers were delivered, we would all get pedicures together and go out to lunch. Katherine and Peggy loved spending time with Caroline, my first baby. They spoiled her and bought her everything. When Katherine and Peggy weren't in town, Jane was spoiling her, keeping her overnight, accompanying me to pediatrician visits, where I would tear up every time she had to get a shot.

Our lives had started to move on. I was able to concentrate on being a mother more than taking care of one. I still handled all her monthly bills, which were high, but that wasn't near the level of work I had done for years before that. After she had lost her teeth and started regressing to her childhood, I decided that the Aricept, which was supposed to slow the progression of her disease, was not helping and was no longer worth the $350.00 a month price tag. When I approached the nurses' station to ask them to discontinue this medicine, they agreed, but then pleaded, "Oh, that's fine. But, whatever you do PLEASE don't stop her Zoloft! If it gets too expensive, we'll take up a collection and help you pay, but please, please, don't make her stop taking it!" I just laughed. So, she wasn't just irritable around me, it was everyone. And they had a hard time imagining how mean she could get if she wasn't on her Zoloft. I agreed to keep her on it as long as she lived.

The next time Cypress Manor showed up on my Caller ID was not about diapers. While we laugh about the story now, it was sad at the time because it led to my mom's last and saddest move.

As I described, Cypress Manor was situated far back from the road, in a lovely setting. The driveway from the main road (a very busy street right off the interstate) to the building must have been at least a quarter of a mile. On this particular morning, one of the Cypress Manor employees found my mother walking down the driveway towards the road. But not just that. She was pushing another woman who was in a wheelchair! A woman she had never met before.

As the employee approached them, she asked, "Where are you two ladies going?"

"We're going out to lunch in Metairie," my mom stated matter-of-factly, as if nothing was wrong with that.

Now I don't have any memory of my mom ever going out to lunch in Metairie, so I have no idea where this thought came from. But the important fact was, not only had she gotten out of the facility, she had taken another resident with her. We were so thankful that someone caught them before they got to the road. There's no telling what could have happened to them.

But this type of behavior is what gets a resident moved to UNIT 3! (Insert ominous background music here.) We knew there was a Unit 3, but we had never been there and had really not given it much thought. Until we were forced to. We were asked to come in that day.

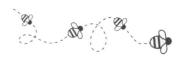

Jane and I entered the office to meet with the administrators. In order for mom to stay at Cypress Manor, she would have to be moved to Unit 3 for her own safety, as well as the safety of the other residents. We were informed that Unit 3 remains locked from the inside and the outside. The doors can only be opened by entering an access code. We would be given an access code which we could use when visiting her, but we could not take her out with us when we left.

They then went on to say that all rooms in Unit 3 were two person rooms. Mom would have a roommate. We were so upset. She had lost her independence and now she would lose her privacy. Who would she be placed with? What condition would they be in? We were already upset when they took us to see what would soon be her new room.

As we walked down the corridors of Units 1 and 2, suddenly they didn't seem so bad. In fact, the people seemed brighter and happier that day. I could picture them watching Aaron's solo Metallica concert. I wished mom had not taken that lady down the driveway.

Our escort led us to a door at the end of a hallway, away from the nurses station in the middle. She stopped and tapped some numbers on a keypad. A green light appeared and we heard a click. She opened the door to Unit 3.

It seemed darker than the rest of the nursing home. Patients were wandering around like ghosts or zombies, walking to nowhere, their faces staring into nothing. What were they thinking about? Some sat in slumped over in wheelchairs in hallways or the common area, wherever they decided to stop moving and nap. As we walked down the hallway, we could hear moaning from other rooms as well as random nonsensical mumbling from others.

The employees were kind to us. They took us to the room mom had been assigned to. At that time, there was not another resident assigned to that room. Whew! No roommate for now. But they assured us there could be one at any time.

The room was slightly larger than her current one. It had two twin beds, two built-in dressers, two closets, and one bathroom. The lady was explaining to us where we could put Mom's chair and TV when Jane and I heard footsteps behind us.

A tall, gaunt, ghost of a man, with a blank expression on his unshaven face, dressed in nothing but a bathrobe, walked into the room, right past where we were standing and into the bathroom. He did not turn on a light or close a door behind him. Next we could hear him urinating in what would be my mom's toilet. Then, without flushing or washing his hands, he walked out the same way he had come in.

We were absolutely horrified. Our mom was going to be in a room where strange men could just walk in half dressed and do whatever they want! Then we heard another strange sound. A woman with a walker was walking the same path, up and down the hallway, mumbling to herself, the same words over and over, just repeating an expletive, not aimed at anyone in particular.

Up the hall and down the hall, constantly, with every other step, "Fucking bitch, fucking bitch, fucking bitch..." She had not stopped by the time we had left and who knows how long or how often she kept up this routine.

As quickly as we could, we gathered Mom's clothes and things and carried them to the new room. We put them away and placed a few family pictures on her nightstand. As her memory faded, we minimized the number of things in her room. We didn't want anything lost or taken and she no longer recognized anything anyway. We left her stuffed animals—mostly tigers—which she liked to hold when she sat in her chair. The employees would have the chair moved so we didn't have to carry that.

Mom was brought into the room and accepted the change without argument. She didn't know she was to be locked in. For her, it wasn't much different and seemed about the same as what she had been used to. For Jane and me, Unit 3 was a nightmare.

We left in a daze, speechless. Then, as we walked to the car, I blurted, "I'm so sure Lurch from *The Addams Family* just walks through the room and pees while we're standing right there!"

And with that, we both burst out laughing. Though we were so sad about mom; throughout this whole ordeal, we had to make jokes and laugh about everything in order to survive.

The laughter was short. We felt horrible. I felt like Mom was going to hate me. I thought I must be the worst daughter ever born if I could leave my mother in that lock-down unit, as I now referred to Unit 3. I couldn't seem to move past the guilt, and it was leading to depression. Not just for me, but for all my sisters.

Finally, Jane and I decided to pay a visit to our favorite pastor, George Haile. This is the man who was the first to hug me after the death of my brother and my dad, who was in the waiting room with us during every surgery described in this book. This man knew my mom as she used to be, the woman in charge of the Sunday School Christmas parties and the Wednesday night suppers. He was now retired, but he agreed to meet with us in his home.

His wife kindly greeted us at the door and showed us to the living room to sit down. She then offered freshly baked homemade coffee cake. My stomach was churning from nerves, but it was impolite to turn it down. Plus, it ended up being really good.

We began explaining everything we had done to take care of our mother. From the first move to Southside Gardens apartments to the lock down in Unit 3. We talked about our guilt and sadness and asked if we were doing the wrong thing. The retired pastor began to speak earnestly to us.

"Girls, in my career, I have witnessed people lose loved ones to everything from accidents to long, drawn-out illnesses. I have presided over funerals for children and people over a hundred years old. I have visited the sick in the hospitals. I have seen a lot of death and comforted many over the loss of a loved one. But, I have to say, in all my years, I have not visited a sadder place than Unit 3."

"Oh no," I began to think.

"But," he continued, "it becomes necessary for some people to be kept there for their own safety and the safety of others. What you need to know is that your mother is not and could not ever be mad at you for the things you've done to care for her. The Mildred Evans we all knew and loved is no longer with us. That's why this disease is so devastating. I call it 'a living death' because the person you love is gone from this world and only a body is left behind, alive, but not there."

"It IS like a living death." I agreed. I kept thinking about Lurch and the lady walking up and down the hall muttering expletives and all the other residents in Unit 3. I remember thinking they all resembled zombies. They were the living dead. Jane and I were both crying by this time.

"One day, your mother's body will go, but her mind and spirit have already gone. Rest assured, she is okay. You girls are suffering way more than she is at this point. She is not aware of what kind of place she is staying in. But you are, so you feel guilt. I'm telling you to let go of that guilt. Your mother is not that body in Unit 3. Your mother is the same woman we all knew and loved, and she is not mad at you; in fact she is grateful for all you have done to take care of her."

"But, her friends...sometimes they act like they are upset with us, like they think we're doing the wrong thing."

"It is hard for her friends to let go of her. They want to think she's still in that body as well. But, she's not. And you girls are the ones who have to deal with her care, and your decisions are perfectly fine. I promise."

"Hmmm. A living death. That makes so much sense," Jane said, wiping a tear.

We finished our coffee cake and tea and caught up on everything else going on in our lives before saying our goodbyes.

After that it was easier to visit Unit 3. We still took turns delivering diapers and visiting Mom. She no longer called us by name, but her eyes showed some signs that she recognized us. I don't think she knew we were her daughters. But she enjoyed the company, so we continued to go.

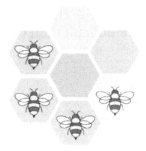

50

IN 2007, I GAVE birth to my second daughter, Katherine Margaret, who goes by "Kate." Now I had two girls named after all four of the Bees: Caroline (my middle name) Jane and Katherine Margaret (Peggy's first name). The tradition of the Four Bees would carry on to the next generation. Also, I could probably score more free babysitting by naming my daughters after all of my sisters.

I know I brought Kate to Cypress Manor at least once because I have a picture. Unit 3 did have one door leading to the outside. It was a closed-in courtyard. The residents were allowed to enjoy some fresh air, trees, birds, and flowers, but could not escape the Unit. We had taken Mom to a seating area in the courtyard and there, I have a picture of her holding Kate when she was a tiny newborn. My mom could not quit staring at her while Kate gripped her index finger and held on tight. Holding my babies always made her happy. I'm not sure she knew she was their grandmother, but I like to think she felt a connection.

With two daughters under two, I was now going to Sam's more often to load up on diapers. I remember how embarrassed I felt running into a friend from high school. I was maneuvering one of the giant carts, the ones they use for large rugs or mattresses.

Only my cart was loaded with as many Pampers Newborn Swaddlers, Huggies Toddler Pull-Ups, and adult pull-up diapers as would fit on the cart. At least I was only in charge of changing two out of the three. I have a special appreciation for the caregivers at nursing homes who change and bathe the residents. It must be so much more difficult than changing a baby.

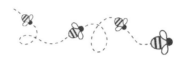

By 2008, we were used to Mom being in lock-down. We still visited with her when we dropped off new supplies of diapers, but she didn't seem to recognize us. Oh, her face lit up when we came into her room, but I think she was just excited to have visitors. Sometimes it seemed like she knew we were somehow related to her or that she was supposed to know us; however, she didn't call us by name. She actually had very little to say and mostly sat quietly in her chair.

In July that year, Charlotte got married. We all got to go to New York City for the wedding, excluding my mother, for obvious reasons. My mother-in-law stayed with my girls in Baton Rouge so I was able to enjoy the grown-up trip to the city. The wedding events were spaced out over enough time that everyone was able to explore on their own. The Bees threw Charlotte a mani/pedi party at a salon on the Upper East Side. Elizabeth designed T-shirts and invitations and we served breakfast and mimosas while all the female wedding guests got their toes and fingers done.

Of course, Peggy pulled out all the stops when it came to her only daughter's wedding. It was at the Boathouse in Central Park. The weather was perfect. Every detail was just right, down to the Pottery Barn keepsake frames holding the place cards at the reception. Tim got up to give a toast and thanked his siblings and family for coming all the way to New York for the wedding and for all they had done to help make the day perfect, then toasted the bride and groom.

In typical Queen Bee style, I approached him afterwards, "I believe you left the most important person out of your speech."

"What do you mean? Who?" He sincerely didn't know what I was talking about.

"Who has been working on this wedding for a year? Who made sure all of this is so perfect? None of this would be happening without her and you didn't even mention her or thank her!"

"Oh, you mean Peggy?"

"Ummmm, yeah! You thanked the whole world except your wife, who did all the work to make this happen!"

As he walked back to the microphone, I thought he would just say he forgot to thank the most important person, without whom we wouldn't be there, and say some wonderful words about Peggy. Instead, he picked up the microphone and explained to the entire room how and why we became known as the Four Bees and that I was the Queen Bee! And as Queen Bee, I had pointed out his mistake and so now he had to apologize. I was so embarrassed, but I supposed I had that coming to me.

When we weren't attending wedding events, we got to go running on the Brooklyn Bridge. I went to the top of Rockefeller Center with Katherine and Cotty. We ate steaks at Peter Luger's, and rode the wooden escalators up every floor of Macy's. We did so much in such a quick time and it was a wonderful trip.

I came home to celebrate Kate's first birthday, giving her a baby doll I bought at F.A.O. Schwartz on the trip.

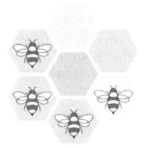

51

IN EARLY SEPTEMBER 2008, Baton Rouge was hit by Hurricane Gustav. By sparing New Orleans, the storm did not garner much national attention, at least not like Katrina or Rita in 2005. But for Baton Rouge, Gustav was devastating. We rode out the storm in our house. The roar of the wind gusts was deafening, but the scariest sound was the popping and snapping which came moments before a tree would fall. Our neighborhood was filled with old water oak trees. Looking out through the windows, I could see the large circles of earth surrounding the tree trunks move as they loosened from the ground with each gust. Then, when the crackling sounds began, I knew it was just moments before one of these trees would fall. The wind lifted trees completely out of the ground and dropped them, leaving root balls standing vertically at least twice my height. Fortunately, the trees in and around our yard fell on our fences, pool, and across roads, rather than on top of our house. Others were not so lucky.

We were without power for over three weeks. Cypress Manor had emergency backup generators, so the residents there were fine. But for a mom of one- and two-year-old girls, this was tragic. With no way to keep milk cold or warm a bottle, bathing or changing diapers in candlelight, and the extreme heat and humidity of post storm south Louisiana, I was desperate by the second day.

As quickly as I could, I packed as many clothes for me and the girls as I could find in the dark. I then loaded them in my car and began driving to stay with Katherine at Cotty's lake house near Johnson City, Tennessee. Katherine agreed to meet me halfway and pick us up at the house of a camp friend in Birmingham. I drove from Baton Rouge to Tuscaloosa, Alabama without stopping for gas, food, or the bathroom. I couldn't make it any further. After filling up with gas, I went to a McDonald's with an indoor playground. I had to pee so bad, I thought I might explode. With Kate in my arms and Caroline's hand in mine, I led them to the McDonald's bathroom. Caroline waited patiently while I stood in the stall wondering how I was going to do this. Although she was over one year old, Kate was not yet walking. I hesitated as long as I could and then, when I could not hold it any longer, I set my baby on the floor of a McDonald's bathroom. Gross! But what else could I do? I peed for what seemed like ten minutes, then scrubbed all of our hands as hard as possible. Then I sat at a table in the play area while they picked at their food and burned some energy off crawling through the tunnels and down the slide.

By the time we made it to Birmingham, I felt so disgustingly dirty I couldn't stand it. I showered and put the girls to bed, then chatted for a while, catching up with my friend and my sister. The next morning, we took off in Cotty's big conversion van to Johnson City. This was much better. The girls were more comfortable and had a TV to watch in the back. I was finally clean and not covered in sweat from lack of air conditioning. When we arrived, I had to make a Target stop first. In my haste, I forgot to pack a stroller, bottles, diapers, wipes, and several other essentials, including beer. When the cashier asked for my ID for the beer, she read my license and saw I was from Louisiana.

"Oh, we were so worried about y'all when that storm was coming, but thank God! It missed New Orleans! You must be so relieved." She seemed proud of her knowledge.

"Yes, but it DID hit Baton Rouge and it's bad. That's why I'm all the way up here. But thank you."

Once I made it to the lake house, I never wanted to leave. I was there for three weeks. In the evenings, I sometimes needed a jacket because it was cool. That would never happen in Louisiana. Katherine took great care of my girls and me, and we got to enjoy a mini vacation with boat rides, lounging on floats in the lake, and even field trips to Blowing Rock, North Carolina, Grandfather Mountain, and Rock City.

After three weeks of being away, I was glad to get home. Although there was debris to be moved and there were insurance claims to be filed, at least we had air conditioning and lights. Things were slowly getting back to normal. I visited Mom at Cypress Manor and it seemed as if nothing had even happened. They had safely weathered the storm and the generators kept everything going until the power was restored. I delivered diapers as usual and paid a visit to my mom. Once again, she was happy for the company, but not sure who I was, and just sat quietly in her chair.

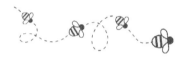

By the first weekend in October, things in Baton Rouge were close to normal. Jane even had power—her neighborhood lost it longer than mine and she had evacuated to Orange Beach, Alabama, followed by a stay in a hotel in Baton Rouge. On Friday October 3, I had a conference scheduled at the Lauberge Casino and Hotel in Lake Charles, Louisiana. Jane and I always loved to go there, so I asked if she wanted to come with me on Thursday and stay through the conference.

We left early Thursday morning, in time to spend the day in the lazy river outside the hotel. After a long day in the sun, we showered, dressed, and headed down to the casino for some fun. We had dinner at one of the hotel restaurants, then split up to play different slot machines. Neither of us was particularly lucky that night, so we went to sleep and decided to try again on Friday.

During my breaks from my classes the next day in the conference center, I would venture over to the casino and find Jane, usually in front of a *Wheel of Fortune* slot machine.

"This is the last time I'm playing," she declared, "I'm leaving in five minutes. I'm going to go to Target and I'll come back when your class is out so we can go home."

Then, I'd come back on my lunch break and see her in the exact same spot in front of the same machine.

"That five minutes lasted over two hours!" I laughed.

She laughed too. "No really, this time I'm leaving. I'm going to Target!"

I said, "Okay, have fun." Then I found a machine and played until the lunch break was over.

When the conference was done for the day, I found her again at the same machine and burst out laughing. "How was Target?"

Her face reddened, "I never went. I've been here all day! It's time to get out of here!"

We loaded up the car and headed back to Baton Rouge. On the way home, she mentioned that Jack had a cross-country meet the following morning and asked if I would like to go. I said yes, thinking it would be good to watch him run, as well as let the girls burn off some energy in the park all morning.

When I dropped her off, she said, "Remember, the meet is at 7:30. If you don't feel like getting up that early on a Saturday, I understand."

"No. I said I was going and I'm going to be there. I'm excited about it." I dropped her off and headed home.

52

THE MORNING OF SATURDAY October 4, 2008, I was still in bed when my cell phone started ringing at 7:20 a.m.

"Oh shit!" I thought when I saw Jane's name on the caller ID. "I'm leaving here in five minutes! I'm getting dressed right now!" I told her, trying hard not to sound like I just woke up.

"We're not going to the cross-country meet," she said.

"What? Why not?"

"Cypress Manor called. Mom is in the hospital."

"What?" I think at some point I got so tired of the calls I told the administration to call Jane first and then me.

"They said they checked on her this morning and she had fallen out of her bed and was lying on the floor. They checked her vitals and her oxygen levels were low so they took her to the emergency room at the Lake." IT was the same hospital where my dad died.

"Okay, I'll get dressed and meet you there."

I showered and dressed for the day. This was becoming routine. I had memorized the smells and sounds of that hospital. And the temperature. I grabbed an extra jacket. Remembering how long my mom lay there after falling at the alumni center with a hole in her lower lip, I was ready for a long day.

I found a parking spot and entered the busy emergency room. Approaching the desk at the end of the waiting area, I explained I was there for Mildred Evans and was shown inside to her room. Of course, in the ER, it wasn't really a room. It was more like a curtained-off booth. She was lying quietly on a bed.

Before I could approach her, I was given a stack of forms to sign. I guess Cypress Manor had given my name as the responsible party when they brought her there. I was surprised that no one from Cypress Manor was with her. Did they really just take their Unit 3 lock-down dementia patients to the emergency room and drop them off alone and unsupervised before a family member even arrived?! I made a mental note to complain about this later.

When I was finally able to approach her, I could detect a glimmer of recognition in her eyes.

"How are you feeling?" I asked.

She didn't speak. She just stared upward.

Jane was there now. We just stood there, looking at each other and at my mom. Her eyes looked so clear that day. It was as if they weren't staring at a hospital ceiling. Instead, they looked like they were actually reflecting the clear blue skies of heaven. I wondered what she was seeing.

"Your eyes are so pretty," Jane told her. She seemed to smile.

We gathered chairs and sat with her in the room/booth, trying to block out the busyness of the emergency room going on outside the curtain. Needing a chance to stretch our legs and move around, we took turns going to the coffee shop, cafeteria, or gift shop for small breaks. We called Peggy and Katherine to let them know what was going on.

"Do you think I need to come down there?" Peggy asked Jane.

"I don't know yet. We'll call you after we talk to the doctor."

They both asked if there was anything they could do. We said no. No one had even come to talk to us, explain what was wrong, or what was going on.

The hours went on. I'm not sure how many, four, five? Going stir-crazy from the quiet, Jane and I decided it would be okay to go together to the coffee shop just once.

We took our time. We talked about how just the day before we were at the casino in Lake Charles.

"I swear! Every single time I saw you at that *Wheel of Fortune* machine, you were like, 'I'm leaving! I'm going to Target!' and then I'd go back an hour or two later and you were still sitting at the same damn machine!" I couldn't help but laugh.

Jane was laughing too. "I know! I really WAS going to Target. Then I would just have to try ONE MORE TIME. Ugh! I should have left."

"Yeah. But we had fun."

"I know. I wish we were still there."

"Me too. This would be a perfect day in that lazy river."

We sipped our lattes from the CC's coffee shop in the hospital and slowly made our way back to the emergency room.

As we approached the check in desk, the same lady who had ushered me back earlier told us to wait there. Then she got up and disappeared into the back. She returned shortly with a man in scrubs, a doctor.

"Are you two here for Mildred Evans?"

"Yes."

"I'm so sorry. She passed away. You can follow me." He brought us back to her room/booth, which was now closed and our chairs had been moved to the outside of the curtain.

"I'm so sorry. There was nothing we could do. Please have a seat here. Our social worker and chaplain are on their way to talk to you and help you through the arrangements."

What? Just like that? It was so strange. I had been notified of death before, but nothing felt like this. I was numb, speechless. So was Jane. For some reason, we didn't cry. We just sat in the chairs.

I tried so hard to feel something. But I couldn't. Could it be relief? No, that would be bad. Was I sad? I was sad for my mom's body, but it had been so long since I had really felt her spirit. Any feeling I had seemed to be wrong, so I just pushed the feelings away.

"It's going to be a long day." I said and Jane agreed.

The social worker came. She was there to help us with the grieving process as well as with the paperwork I would need to review and sign. Did she think we were bad daughters because we were not crying? I started signing pages, choosing the funeral home to which they could have the body sent.

We needed to start calling people. Notifying friends and family. We needed to make arrangements and find George Haile. Now retired, he was the only person we would allow to perform the service. Jane tried to get in touch with him. I notified Peggy.

"Do you think I need to come down there?" The same question as earlier, but this time a decision was necessary.

"Yes, Peggy. You need to come down here."

Then I called Katherine. Bitch Number 2.

"Mom just died."

Without missing a beat, she replied, "Well, at least she did it on the open date."

MIC DROP!

This has to be one of the fastest, funniest, and most timely lines she has ever come up with. I thought about the rule for weddings in the south: ALWAYS PLAN AROUND THE FOOTBALL SCHEDULE. It was the perfect Mildred Evans way to exit! That Saturday, LSU had a "bye week" and no one would be missing any football, home or away, on her account! After all the years she spent working and volunteering for the school she loved, it was so like her to do this.

Also, I believe she chose to wait for Jane and me to leave the room together, just like my dad waited for everyone but Mom to leave his hospital room. I don't think she wanted one of us to be alone with her when it happened, so she just held on. Staring up at heaven, having it reflected in her eyes, waiting for us to get our coffee so she could move on by herself.

By the time Jane was off of the phone and I told her what Katherine had said, we were both giggling so hard we had tears by the time the chaplain showed up. Little did he know they were tears from laughter. We tried so hard to stifle our amusement and make the tears seem grief-driven as he sat and prayed with us. I'm sure he and the social worker thought we were cold-hearted or just mean. It's just that sometimes, especially times of stress, my humor comes to the surface while my sadness tries to suppress itself underneath.

Jane finally got in touch with George Haile. He was out of town and would not be available to do the service until Wednesday. It was going to be a long five days, but we had to wait. There would be no one else capable of handling this for us.

We did venture behind the curtain for one look. The body was cold, empty. Eyes closed, lifeless, small, my mother's spirit long gone. I didn't look for long. That was not her. Not really. In my mind, she was finally embracing Red, the love of her life, and her daddy, her mama, and her baby son, Jack. A joyous family reunion that we were not invited to, at least not yet.

With all the paperwork done and most of our phone calls made, we left the hospital and headed downtown to Rabenhorst Funeral Home, where my brother's funeral and Dad's visitation had been.

53

WHILE I HAD BEEN there with my mother to plan arrangements for my dad, I had not been in charge of the business of planning a funeral before. It's such a peculiar venue and situation. Walking in, everything is mortally quiet. Telling the greeter who we were and why we were there, I felt compelled to whisper.

We were led to an office and seated while the director brought out more paperwork for me. We would be responsible to write an obituary, which they would arrange to publish in the local paper and online. (I made a mental note to put Peggy in charge of this.) They would furnish us with five certified copies of the death certificate, included in the price of the funeral, but we would have to pay extra if we wanted more. We could furnish pictures which could be played on a computer screen during visitation, if we wished, for a fee.

There was so much business that went into the planning of a funeral. It was hard to imagine how these people managed to keep an attitude of condolence while presenting their products and packages like car salesmen. Of course, it's got to be easier than selling a car. The customer has just lost someone dear to them and their mind is not exactly ready to wheel and deal on the price of a slideshow.

Next, we were led into a large room of caskets to choose one for my mother. I remembered how my brother and father were laid in plain wooden caskets with little in the way of adornments. I knew my mom would want the same. Nothing fancy or silver or pink. Walking in I pointed to the first plain wooden one I saw that looked similar.

"We'll take that one," I pointed to it, proud of my quick decisiveness.

"How large of a woman was your mother?" the director asked.

"Oh, well she lost a lot of weight in the last few years. And she shrank from her osteoporosis. I'd guess probably around 5'2", maybe 90-100 pounds."

"Well, you have selected one of our enhanced sizes," (maybe funeral speak for XXL?) "Can I direct you to choose one from this wall over here for something more appropriate for her?"

"Oh. Sure." I didn't know caskets came in sizes. Nobody ever told me that. Except that I had seen the baby and child ones across the room. Otherwise, I thought a casket was a casket.

I went to the wall he pointed me to and selected the plain wooden one in the correct size. There. That's done.

"Now, what cemetery do you plan to use?"

This one was easy. "She already has a plot next to my father and brother at Resthaven." Whew. At least that was already paid for and arranged.

"Okay, I'll call them and let them know you are coming. Can you meet with them tomorrow morning?" Meet with them? Why did they need to meet?

"Alright. Just let me know what time."

He led me back to the office, where he presented the final bill for more than ten thousand dollars. I wrote him a check and got out of there as fast as I could. I felt dirty. And tired. And emotionally confused and drained.

"I need a beer. How about you?" I asked Jane.

She agreed and we headed to a barbecue place nearby and sat down with cold bottles of beer to begin to process the day. Other football teams were playing on the TV screens surrounding the restaurant and I couldn't help but laugh and be glad that we weren't missing an LSU game. "Thanks, Mom." I told her silently.

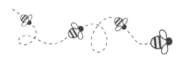

After leaving the restaurant, I returned home, exhausted. What had started out as me thinking I was late for my nephew's cross-country meet had turned into one of the longest days of my life. I still hadn't cried. I still wasn't sure what to feel. I just knew I was tired. I hugged my girls and put them to bed and fell asleep, dreamless.

The following morning, Jane and I had to drive out to Resthaven, the cemetery, to meet with the director. By now, Peggy and Katherine were on their way to Baton Rouge and relatives and friends had been notified about my mother's passing. It was just a matter of getting the arrangements organized and paid for by Wednesday. It was only Sunday. This was going to be a long week.

We walked into the Resthaven facility and, like the funeral home, it was quiet. I felt as if we had to whisper. I was tired. I was ready to get this over with. What did we really need to do here anyway? The plot was paid for. Wasn't that all they needed? I still had a lot to learn about funeral planning and costs.

We were seated across the desk from the manager who had some files stacked on the desk in front of him. He started by greeting us.

"Good morning. I'm so sorry for your loss."

"Thank you," we each replied and introduced ourselves.

He began describing different types of vaults underground which held the casket. I didn't know this existed. I just thought the casket was buried in the dirt.

"Well, we have the plain one-layer concrete vault, which will run around $4,000."

I gulped. *There's still more to pay for?!* I thought, wondering how much money my mother had left and whether I was going to have to find a way to handle this.

"Of course, the more secure vaults are lined and can run up to $12,000." His voice began to trail off as he described the different underground vaults and their prices. What were these things? Were they really necessary?

"We'll take the $4,000 plain concrete one." I spoke decisively.

"Hmmm. I assumed you would probably make that choice. Prior to our appointment, I took the liberty of pulling the file from your father's funeral. It seems your mom chose the (insert name of the super-duper, most expensive vault here) for your father. I figured if she wanted it for him, she would probably want the same for herself."

What!? I was thinking to myself, *This guy is trying the hard upsell on me when my mom died yesterday! And he's dropping the guilt on me—trying to tell me what my mom would want.* I was beginning to think funeral homes and cemeteries were just death versions of used car lots.

"We're going to stick with the $4,000 choice. Thank you so much for your time and research."

I couldn't get out of there fast enough.

Back at home, it was time to rest and wait. We needed to gather pictures for the slide show and for a giant photo board that my neighbor was making to display on an easel in the funeral home. (He worked for a company which created exhibits for lawyers to use in jury trials.) Peggy was working on the obituary and would turn it in to the funeral home when she got into town. For now, we just needed to get through the next three days and it would be over.

On Monday, we all had errands to do, but we planned a Bees visit to the nail place to get pedicures and manicures. Not so much because we needed pretty nails for the funeral, but because it would be fun to hang out together and relax.

Before we headed out for errands, Peggy asked in her softest, sweetest voice, "Virginia, what do you need me to do to help?"

"Can you go to Cypress Manor and get Mom's blue St. John knit dress and drop it off at the funeral home?"

"Oh sure, I can do that."

"Thank you so much. That will be a huge help."

I can't remember where everyone else had to go. The reception after the service would be held at Jane's house. She had so many friends who always stepped up to help in any kind of situation, so they were handling the food and drinks, as well as keeping a list of what people were dropping off. People always bring food or something to the house when there's going to be a funeral.

My mother-in-law would be coming into town to keep my girls during the service so I wouldn't have to chase a one- and a two-year-old all over the funeral home and cemetery. But I was still caring for them on that Monday and Tuesday as well as trying to get my house ready for company from out of town.

It was several hours before I made it to Jane's that afternoon to meet up for our trip to the nail place. Peggy had not yet returned from her single errand. We just waited patiently. There was no hurry, as we still had two days to go before this would be over.

Eventually, Peggy walked through the door to Jane's kitchen carrying several bags from Dillard's, a department store in the mall. She carefully emptied the contents of the bags and spread them out on Jane's kitchen table.

"Virginia, I wasn't sure what size bra mother wore so I picked three for you to choose from. I also bought her several pairs of underwear because I didn't know what kind she liked. Then, I couldn't decide on which color panty hose she would want to wear with the blue dress, so I bought three pairs. You can decide which ones she would like, and I can return the rest to Dillard's."

Now, I know her heart was in the right place and her intentions were good. She wanted to help, to contribute to the work and planning that was going into this funeral. But something in that moment made me snap. All the feelings that I had not felt since Saturday morning came bubbling up from deep inside me. As calmly as possible I stated, firmly, "I'm letting you all know right now: if and when I die, if ANYBODY tries to bury me in panty hose, I will absolutely come back and haunt you for the rest of your life! And I don't care what bra or underwear Mom wears. She's getting buried. She doesn't know or care!" Then, storming out of the door, I turned and said, "Y'all have fun at the nail place, I'm done. I'm going home."

I know it was so mean. I should not have acted like that. But at that moment, everything in front of me was a blur. I knew I was about to lose all control and release every feeling I had been holding back. I needed to get home to my room, and fast.

I threw myself on my bed and sobbed. I rocked back and forth on my hands and knees, crying out, "I want my mom!" She was the only one who could comfort me at that moment and she was gone. And I didn't want the mom who had died two days ago. I wanted the mom of my childhood, the one who wrote letters to me at camp, the one who made sure I always had the perfect dress for every occasion, and the one who would have hugged and comforted me when I was grieving. A living death. I finally mourned the loss of my mother's body as well as her brain.

I begged her to forgive me for feeling relief that her body had died. I acknowledged to her and to myself that I had been missing her for years and that caring for that body was a painful chore. Did she understand that? Did she know how much it hurt every time I went to visit, or brought diapers, or had to move her, or take her car? Did she know that it hurt me more than it hurt her? And now I was finally releasing it. The jokes were funny and had sustained us through the years, but now I recognized how much pain was beneath that laughter.

"If I ever get like that, lock me up in a nursing home and forget about me! I'm serious! Don't even visit me."

Her words came back to me yet again. She understood. It killed her to see her mother forget everyone and everything only to become someone my mom didn't recognize. She did not wish that on us.

I knew her mind and body were now reconnected and she was at peace, embracing her loved ones as she looked down on her Four Bees, now as a guardian angel.

I cried softly in the bed until I fell asleep. Later, after waking up, I called to apologize to my sisters for my outburst. There were no hard feelings. They had gotten their manicures and pedicures. Peggy had chosen some undergarments to deliver to the funeral home with the blue dress from Cypress Manor. Now we just had to get through two more days.

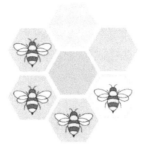

54

AFTER SOLIDIFYING MY POSITION as Bitch Number 1 by throwing a tantrum and skipping the spa day, I woke up Tuesday ready to act like a grown-up again. I got my own manicure and pedicure and further straightened my house in case out-of-town company would be coming in.

Peggy had turned in the obituary, which was beautifully written. She had so many details about my mom's life in there that I never would have remembered. She also made sure the funeral home had all the pictures for the slide show on a thumb drive. Jane was busy getting her house ready for the reception following the funeral.

Unbeknownst to me, all of my mom's grandchildren (except mine, who were still babies) were busy writing their memories of my mom, which would be read aloud at the service, along with a story of my mother written by her college roommate and best friend, Dot Howell.

All the arrangements were coming together, now everyone just needed to wait and see if Bill would show up. Peggy had always been the only one to communicate with him, so she had notified him of her death and all the arrangements that had been made.

We weren't anxious about seeing him. In fact, none of us carried any anger for him with us anymore. The fight in the hospital during my mom's aorta surgery, leaving Mom at the alumni center, even the fight in Williamsburg, all seemed a distant memory, even though the nickname stuck and we were still the Four Bees.

When the morning of the funeral arrived, my stomach revolted. I was in the bathroom all morning. I knew it was my nerves and not some sort of virus, but I wanted it gone. I took so much over-the-counter medicine, I probably clogged up my system for a week. I was finally able to get dressed and leave my babies with my mother-in-law and head to the funeral home.

Once there, I noticed that the crowd was much smaller than that at my dad's funeral. It wasn't that my mom didn't have as many friends. If anything, she had more. I realized that so many of their friends had passed away between my dad's death in 1993 and my mom's in 2008. We were losing the Greatest Generation at an alarming rate. Soon, there would be few people in Baton Rouge who would remember Mildred and Red Evans. The people I thought were larger than life would be forgotten and replaced with newer and younger community leaders.

I did notice a great number of my own friends. I was able to pick them out and speak to them. My old law school roommate, Amie, was there and I would use her to sneak away with me any time I needed a break from standing in the line, greeting people I didn't know. It was during one of these outings when I spotted Bill. We ran around the corner and outside the building, giggling like school girls. I had evaded him, even though it was only for a short time.

Soon, music began to play and the service began. People sang hymns, George Haile led everyone in prayer, and then he read the letters from my nieces and nephews and Dot Howell. Hearing these memories was touching and I was just about to tear up when suddenly, from behind me, I heard it. It hadn't changed in all these years. Just as loud and just as obnoxious.

"AHHH-CHAAAWWWW!!!"

When we heard Bill's sneeze interrupt the quiet of the service, all four of us had to bite our lips and squeeze our eyes to keep from laughing out loud. I was holding in so much laughter that my face reddened and tears actually streamed down my face. I hadn't cried all day and now, there I was, crying from laughter in the middle of my mother's funeral. I hope I had pulled off my act and that the guests saw my red face and tears as a show of grief at the loss of my mom.

We made it from the funeral home through the graveside service at the cemetery, then headed over to Jane's house for the reception. Her friends already had everything set out beautifully. I wasn't around to see it, but when Bill walked in and saw Jane he reached out his hand to shake hers.

"Nice to meet you ... I mean, see you." he said.

"Good to see you, too," she replied. And I believe that was the extent of anyone's conversations with him.

Bill had a son around Jack's age and they jumped together on the trampoline in Jane's back yard. My friends and I took turns riding around the neighborhood on Jane's golf cart with Elizabeth and Brittany. My Uncle Charlie sat in a chair in Jane's living room telling story after story as he chain-smoked all afternoon. He would light one cigarette before he had finished putting out the one he just finished. Yet he was the only one of my mom's siblings to live into his 90s and keep his wits about him to the very end.

Eventually, the guests said their goodbyes and filed out. Weary from a day of standing and greeting guests as well as processing my roller coaster of emotions, I was ready to go home and sleep. I couldn't believe it was all over.

Over the next few days, I had Peggy and Katherine go to Cypress Manor and take what few clothes and belongings my mother had and either throw them away or take them to goodwill. Most were ruined from the stale urine smell, and got trashed along with her recliner. I took care of the final bill and signed whatever paperwork was needed to have her checked out. We were done. No more diapers, late-night calls, or visits with not much to say to a mother who didn't even know us. We left Cypress Manor forever in the background.

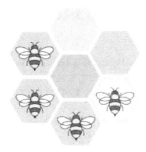

55

I'M NOT SURE WHY I felt such a tremendous pressure on me to be successful or do something special or great. I think that I always looked up to both of my parents with such admiration. I revered everything they had been through in their lives and how they overcame obstacles without fear, moving forward bravely in each phase of their lives. From the Great Depression, murder of a father, World War II, to full careers, raising six children, along with service to church and community. I never thought I was good enough to be their child. They were so perfect. What could I possibly do that could make them proud?

I had started by trying to be an architect or a civil engineer. That was a huge flop. I went to law school and became a lawyer. But I never have loved it the way my father loved his work. I am a mother of two beautiful daughters, but sometimes I feel like I've made so many mistakes with them and our relationship is nothing like what I had with my parents growing up. Why have I always felt like I'm not good enough?

In 2011, I was being interviewed for a job when I was asked the question.

"Name a situation or obstacle that was particularly challenging to you. What steps did you take to handle it and how did you overcome it?"

I sat for at least a minute then asked, "Does it have to pertain to law or work?"

"No, it can be any challenge you have overcome."

The answer that came to me was perfectly clear.

"I was the youngest of six children. We were spread out over 22 years. My parents were 47 and 50 when I was born," I began.

"Wow. Go on."

"I was always the baby of the family. Somewhat spoiled. My father passed away in 1993. A few years later, my mom developed Alzheimer's disease."

"Oh. I'm so sorry."

"Even though I was the youngest, I somehow became 'in charge' of her care. I had to take her keys away when she could no longer drive, even though I knew that would make her despise me. I drove her to doctor appointments and hair appointments. Later, I had to move her and sell her home. I would end up moving her through four levels of care facilities. Eventually, I would plan her funeral.

I became like the oldest child. I was a primary caregiver for my mother while running a title company and caring for two babies of my own. And looking back, even though it was difficult and heartbreaking at times, I believe that was one of my greatest accomplishments."

The lady agreed that I had overcome a great challenge. She called a few days later and offered me the job; however, I had already accepted another position by then. But I have to think my answer to that one question played a part in my getting the offer.

Answering that question helped me in so many ways. Maybe I was good enough. I too could face challenging circumstances and have the courage to overcome them and come out better for it. I could be successful in life without having the best career or a collection of accolades for all my achievements. My success could be measured by choosing love, laughter, family, and gratitude despite the obstacles which life would throw in my path.

.

Epilogue

MY MOTHER HAS BEEN gone almost thirteen years. I have lived on this earth longer without my dad than I have with him. Where did all that time go?

Since my mom's funeral, the Four Bees have been through what seems like another full lifetime of major milestones:

Foreclosures
Job loss (personal and close family members)
Divorces
House burned down
Remarriages
Death of a child
Illness of a child
Parental alienation
Motorcycle crash
New marriages
New children
Retirements
New jobs
Global Pandemic

Along with more than one bout with alcoholism, depression, anxiety, ADHD, or a combination of conditions.

Through the strength of our sisterhood, we've been able to help each other get up and live our best lives, even when we thought we had finally hit rock bottom. Even when we got knocked down to a lower rock bottom.

And you know what I've learned? I think you need to hit some rock bottoms to really live this life of ours. If you haven't been hurt, really hurt, then you can't get back up and try again. You learn to appreciate so much more of this wonderful world. To be grateful for the new day, the sun, flowers, music, a smile, the touch of a loved one, the voice of a friend, family, and sisters. These are the important things, and if I can have these, I am successful. If I had to hit rock bottom to learn this, then it was worth it. I have these. I am grateful. I am successful. And my parents are proud.

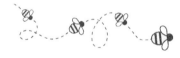

I don't remember exactly what year I began to host Thanksgiving annually at my house. It was after Aaron's second son, Isaac, was born. I remember that because the first time they came, Isaac was still in a high chair and he passed out face-down in his food right in the middle of Thanksgiving dinner.

The idea sort of caught on. Tim realized, "Wow, Thanksgiving is pretty fun in Baton Rouge at Virginia's!" For the first time, I think he began to look forward to his annual trip to be with his in-laws. The next year, Charlotte and her husband came to Baton Rouge from New York to join in the fun. Each year it has grown and now it has solidified as a reunion of the Bees and a ritual to carry on the traditions started by Mildred and Red many years ago.

Everyone usually begins arriving in town by Wednesday, and stays through Sunday. In our family, Thanksgiving is considered a marathon, not a sprint. Wednesday night, I usually serve seafood gumbo, which can be served as people arrive and not at any particular time. So far, we've been blessed with excellent weather. Cool enough, but not too much rain. In the evenings, there's always a fire in the fire pit outside. Aaron, always the Texan, continues to pile wood on top of the fire, keeping it way taller than necessary to keep everyone warm and comfortable. Everyone reunites with hugs and greetings to the children, especially about how much they've grown over the past year. We talk and catch up and plan the events of the rest of the weekend while enjoying drinks around the fire pit.

Sometimes, that Wednesday night ends a little later than it should because the next morning most of us venture downtown before 8:00 a.m. to participate in the annual Turkey Trot. The children usually do the one-mile fun run and the adults run in the 5K. We don't break any records, but I consider it as a way to earn a day of eating and drinking with no guilt.

After the race, everyone splits up and goes about their own activities. Some take the little kids to see Mike the Tiger across from the LSU football stadium. I go home and turn on the Macy's Thanksgiving Day Parade. I do not remember a single Thanksgiving growing up when that parade wasn't on the TV. I loved to see the Rockettes, and of course, Santa Claus. Now I have it on as background noise while I begin to cook.

I don't do everything like Mildred did. That would be impossible. It's not better or worse, just different. I make cornbread dressing in advance and freeze it. My recipe makes so many dirty dishes and takes so much time that it would be impossible for me to do it on Thanksgiving Day along with everything else. Jane makes several sides and brings them early to warm up in my oven. Elizabeth makes my mom's squash casserole. Sometimes Katherine makes one or two of my mom's pie recipes.

The night before Thanksgiving, we inject two turkeys with a Cajun-style injectable marinade. This is also something my mom never did. Then on Thanksgiving Day, we fry one in peanut oil outside in a giant pot over a propane flame. I bake the other one in the oven. I use the drippings to make gravy for the rice and mashed potatoes. Gravy was definitely a learning process. My mom tried teaching it to me when she still had her mind and I do recall some of her "tricks." But I also have added some tricks of my own. And some of Jane's. I always make black-eyed peas and green beans (but not the green bean casserole).

Every year we have to have crescent rolls. When she was little, Brittany always wanted to roll the dough into the crescent shapes. So I would pop open the can and help her place them on the pan as she rolled them. Later, she helped my daughters roll up the crescent rolls. Later when they were older, one of my daughters usually helped one of Aaron's boys, Nathan and Isaac, roll the crescent rolls. It's always been like this and I like that the youngest in the group have some participation role in the family meal. Soon, I'm sure Nathan and Isaac will be helping Charlotte's son, Henry, roll up the crescent rolls. Next will be Brittany's son, Ezra. Life goes on.

My house is much smaller than my mom's was. It's even smaller than the old house before the new addition. But the kitchen is open to the living and dining areas, so everyone can visit during the cooking process. Like I said, we have been blessed so far with good weather. We've been able to set up enough tables outside on my patio for everyone to have a place to sit and enjoy their meal, no matter how large the crowd grows. I think the number is over thirty now, but the more the merrier and I love it.

One of the most important Thanksgiving traditions I carry on is the blessing. I usually call on Tim to say a prayer before the meal is served. Everyone gathers around the kitchen island, where the food is waiting to be served. I usually say a few words first. One year I mentioned that I had put the turkey in the oven at 11:11 a.m. It dawned on me that I had never told my family this, but every time I happen to glance at a clock by accident and it is 11:11, to me it means that my mom is watching over me and she is proud. So I believe that she was proud that day that her family still gathers together from all over the country to share a meal of true Thanksgiving. Tim follows with a prayer thanking God for all of our blessings as well as the food before us. When he couldn't come because of Covid, I had Aaron say the prayer. He was so surprised and honored to have this duty and he delivered it beautifully.

I don't use Lenox holiday china or sterling silver flatware. Another way I'm different from Mildred is I like to have fun after the long day of cooking and that doesn't involve washing thirty sets of dishes. We spring for the good paper plates, strong enough to hold a heavy load of turkey with all the sides piled up as high as one can pile it. We buy the sturdy plastic flatware. I try to even use the disposable foil trays for my sides now so there aren't even as many serving dishes to clean. Not that I don't have help. I do. Especially from Peggy. And Katherine.

After the meal, I like to relax by the fire and enjoy drinks and games with all my family that I only see once a year. It all started when Charlotte's husband brought Cards Against Humanity for the first time. We all laughed until tears were streaming down our faces and our cheeks ached when Tim had to read out loud, "balls deep into a squealing pig!"

Now, we've tried different games but it's always a good time. Except the time we played Buzzed and everyone in the family conspired to make up questions rather than read the ones actually printed on their cards. They decided to only ask questions that would make me have to take a sip of my drink. My nephew had made that drink. And it tasted *gooooood!* But, it must have been strong! I don't remember the last half of the night and have since named his drinks "Mind Erasers" and know to be careful when he's tending the bar.

On the Friday after Thanksgiving, we usually do something to celebrate Jane's birthday. The first year it was bowling. Then we began going to the river house, where she lives now. Her husband has groves of citrus trees and at that time of year they are heavy with satsumas and oranges. The younger kids pluck the fresh fruit from the trees and the older ones operate his industrial size squeezer to make juice, which is then mixed with champagne for homemade mimosas. They have a tip jar set up by the glasses of fresh juice and tend to make out well.

Then Jane's husband takes the kids and the out-of-towners on a party barge ride down the river and through the bayou. It's a slow enjoyable ride, unless they spot an alligator—then it gets a bit more exciting. Everyone comes back and eats chicken, red beans, and birthday cake until it's almost dark. Football is always playing at every house and no matter what, all eyes are glued to the Iron Bowl (Alabama v. Auburn for those who may not be SEC people) and LSU v. Texas A&M.

On the following Saturday, if LSU has a home game, we try to get as many tickets as we can for family members to attend the game. Everyone without a ticket is welcome to watch the game at the tailgate. We tailgate all day long with friends, even more family, food, keg beer, and purple and gold Jell-O shots. It's usually fun for everyone involved...except for the one year when Charlotte was pregnant and sober trying to navigate her drunk husband through Tiger Stadium and find something vegan for him to eat at the concession stand. I guess he had been nagged one time too many times when he looked at her sloppily and demanded that she "Be A Better Person!" The following year, instead of "Happy Birthday Jane," the Chantilly cake Elizabeth brought to Thanksgiving dinner had red icing in cursive spelling out "Be A Better Person." The new Thanksgiving slogan was born.

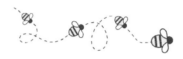

Sometime after he outgrew the high chair, Aaron's youngest son Isaac earned the nickname "Kraken," after the mythical sea monster who wreaks havoc destroying everything in its path. On the Wednesday evening after they arrived, he somehow managed to take a wholesale club-sized jar of Nestle Quik powder and dumped it all over my couches and rug. I believe Peggy and Claire were trying to hastily vacuum up the chocolate mess when he ventured into another room to pour glue on another couch as well as in someone's shoes. Katherine managed to stop him from cutting off all his fingers in a cigar cutter. After that, he managed to turn on the gas to the indoor fireplace (which I didn't even know worked). Luckily, someone smelled it and turned it off as the door to that room was open to the patio where the fire pit was fully blazing with Aaron's Texas sized wood pile. We were all fortunate not to blow up that night.

The next morning, after the Turkey Trot, I went home and turned on the Macy's parade as usual. When I looked up at the television, I was horrified to see that the entire screen had been colored over in markers. I glanced over at a table across the room where my girls had been making place cards for the tables the day before. The table was scattered with a random mixture of washable Crayola markers and permanent Sharpie markers. I was silently praying as I calmly went to the kitchen to grab the Windex and some paper towels. As I started to wipe the TV screen, I gave a big, "Thank You Jesus" when all of the writing wiped off. It's pure luck that that boy only happened to color my television screen with washable markers.

The Kraken has outgrown his nickname by now and is quite a sweet and respectable boy. I'm proud of Aaron and his boys. I'm proud of all of my nieces and nephews. They have earned places in my heart right up there with the Bees. They have taken care of me when I was down and created memories and laughter that I will always treasure. My girls are so fortunate to have each and every one of them as a cousin.

Aaron is a grown-up now. He's much taller than me, with a deep, jolly voice and an outgoing, friendly, contagious personality that seems to spread happiness. He builds swimming pools and is lucky enough to get paid for doing what he loves. He also loves his wife, his boys, and God. He's even been ordained! He seems to have endless energy and is always working on a project. He has the creative gene. He can draw, paint, play guitar, and design and create unique and lovely indoor and outdoor projects around his home. He has a long, long, beard—like ZZ Top long. And I wouldn't want him any other way. One of my all time favorite posts on Facebook was in mid 2020 when Aaron wrote:

"So yesterday after work I went by my local Kroger and visited the meat market as I usually do on Fridays to line up our grillables for the weekend. With the new ordinance in Dallas County coming back around again about masks, I was in there wearing my mask, in compliance.

I've been going to this shop for years and I have lots of friends in the butchers area they have guided me well over the years. This time though it was different they have a new person in there. So the new person said to me, 'Hey you're the Grill Guy right?" I was very thankful that your crew had already informed the person.

So I told the employee, 'Thank you so much, do you have any idea how much meat I buy to not be known as "long beard guy"?'

We had a great laugh for a few minutes and then I headed home to fire up the grill. I don't want this to turn into a debate about wearing masks or not—that part is irrelevant. Share the funny and awesome moments of your day. We need it, and we only pass through this place once, so make it count and share a smile and a laugh; it's so much easier when you do...and more fun."

I couldn't help but smile and love him for this post. Finding the laughter among the chaos. That's what we had to do with my mom's Alzheimer's, and that's what we have to do with life. And it works.

Aaron and his family now live on the North Carolina coast, in Hampstead. I have visited them there and they seem so much happier than they had been in Texas—if you can believe that. They visit the turtle hospital, the beaches, and participate in all sorts of local activities.

Charlotte got the creative gene as well. She has been all over the world with theater degrees from Texas, Harvard, and Scotland. She has acted in plays in New York City and beyond. She has coached others through their careers in theatre. And she has become an accomplished portrait photographer. One of my favorite parts of Thanksgiving is viewing her pictures documenting the weekend. Her latest project is very close to my heart. With help from Peggy and Katherine with the organizing, scanning, and converting to typed documents, she has accumulated all of my parents' letters to each other during World War II. Carefully studying each one, she has learned what they were feeling deep in their souls at that fearful and precious time. Combining their love for one another as expressed through the letters with my mother's scattering and rereading of them throughout her Alzheimer's progression, Charlotte has managed to write an incredible play entitled, *The War Letters*, which I have been to see in New York twice! She also has a podcast, which is a fascinating discussion of the time period of the war at home and abroad, combined with a great appreciation for the art of handwritten communication—something we've lost with the advent of text, email, and social media. Charlotte never gives up on her dreams. She is a true artist and she inspires me to this day.

Elizabeth not only got the creative gene, but she was the first descendant of Red Evans to become an architect. And not just any architect. She graduated with honors from LSU with a Masters in Architecture and received the medal awarded to the best graduate student in the LSU College of Design. She has won several awards and high accolades since then, and had many works featured in the newspaper. She now works for the architect who wrote the moving poem read at my father's funeral. I remember feeling not only a chest full of pride at her graduation, but a little weight lifting off of my shoulders. I had mistakenly believed that I had to do what my dad did in order to make him proud. Now, I knew that was wrong, but I still had a sense of relief that someone in the family was going to do it. Someone would use his drawing table and his instruments. And she does. Sometimes. Of course, most architects use computers to draw now and don't have holes worn through the elbows of all their dress shirts.

Brittany is a first grade teacher and spreads joy, humor, and creativity to all who are lucky enough to be a part of her classroom. She has won several awards for Best Teacher of the Year and has been asked to speak at trainings for other elementary school teachers about the methods she uses in her class. I don't know if it has to do with her methods or if it's just Brittany's personality that makes her so successful. I know I can't be around her without smiling, and she brings her talent selflessly to the most unfortunate children in the Baton Rouge community. She genuinely cares about people and is always a friend to all.

Each year I am so blessed to have this time to spend with the Bees and their families. We grow and we change. People go and new people join us. Now Jane has a home on the Mississippi gulf coast and we will start having some Thanksgiving meals there!

The most important thing to me is that we always stay together no matter where we live or what we are going through. And I can't forget to be thankful for Bill. If it wasn't for him, we wouldn't forever and ever be the Four Bees!

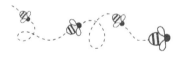

On the Sunday after Thanksgiving, everyone goes home and I just fall down flat, exhausted from the four-day marathon of food, drinks, catching up, and laughing. It's a satisfying kind of tired. I know I will have to decorate for Christmas soon, but not that day. I do still love Christmas and it still reminds me of my mother. I put up a tree and some of her snow village houses. I love buying gifts for everyone and trying to come up with creative surprises. But Thanksgiving is my favorite holiday. I have learned so much about gratitude over the years and what a blessing it is to have something to be thankful for each day on this Earth. Especially family and laughter.

After my girls went back to school, I was driving them home one afternoon. They're thirteen and fifteen now, so Mom is not their favorite person to talk to. But I try to make small talk. As I went through the green light that leads me to our street, I asked, "So, do you have very much homework tonight?"

With a stiff arm crossing and the perfected teen eye roll one of them replied, "MOM! That's the third time you've asked the same question in like the last five minutes! NO! We don't! How do you NOT remember that?"

At over 50 years old, I just grinned as I thought of their future as well as mine. "Buckle up girls. It's going to be a long ride!"

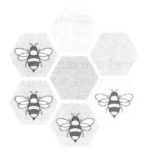

Acknowledgments

I HAVE THE DEEPEST gratitude and appreciation for Peggy, Katherine, and Jane. You have always shown your love and support for me throughout my life. I could not do life without you. Thank you for going through all these experiences with me and for lifting me up when I needed it. I will always love you and be exceptionally grateful to be your little sister.

To Caroline and Kate, when I found out I was having girls my deepest desire was for you to be as close to each other as I am with my sisters. I named you Caroline Jane (after Virginia Caroline Evans and Jane Evans Lundin) and Katherine Margaret (after Katherine Evans and Margaret "Peggy" Evans Purser). I have all of the best hopes and dreams for your future in this life. You each mean the world to me and I will always love you more than you can possibly imagine.

To Charlotte for reading the first draft of this manuscript and providing your feedback, as well as offering to record the audiobook of *The Youngest Bee*. Your play, *The War Letters*, is a beautiful depiction of the love story of Mildred and Red as well as a deeply heartbreaking and inspirational perspective through Mildred's eyes as she became confused, and eventually lost her memory. You are extremely talented and inspire me to want to continue trying to create. Thank you to Elizabeth for your amazing cover design. You have carried on your Granddad's legacy well and we are all proud of you. As an architect, artist, and person you are creative, talented, inspirational, and loving. I can't thank you enough for gracing *The Youngest Bee* with your talents.

I thank those who read through the first manuscript of *The Youngest Bee* and provided your feedback including, but not limited to, Martha Strohschein, Tison Pugh, and Kristin Delahoussaye, as well as my sisters and Charlotte. You are very patient and forgiving with your comments, and I am so grateful for each of you.

Finally to Liz Hill at Green Heart Living Press. If you had not taken a chance on me and agreed to publish this book I don't know that it would ever have gotten out of my laptop and onto paper. I knew we would be a good fit when I first learned that your group of authors was named the "Hive." Our meetings always left me feeling positively inspired, believing that I actually might be able to do this. I appreciate all of your time, coaching, and listening. Thank you for making my dream come true!

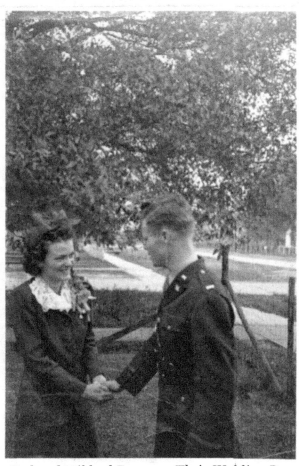

Red and Mildred Evans on Their Wedding Day,
November 28, 1942

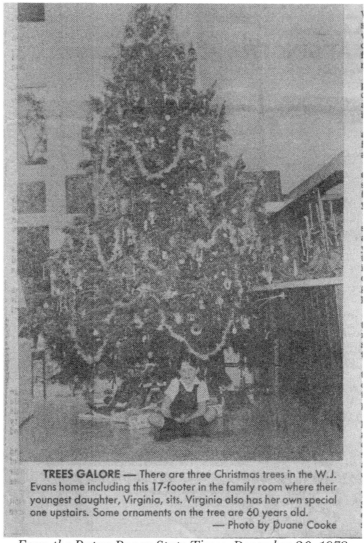

TREES GALORE — There are three Christmas trees in the W.J. Evans home including this 17-footer in the family room where their youngest daughter, Virginia, sits. Virginia also has her own special one upstairs. Some ornaments on the tree are 60 years old.
— Photo by Duane Cooke

From the Baton Rouge State Times, December 20, 1978

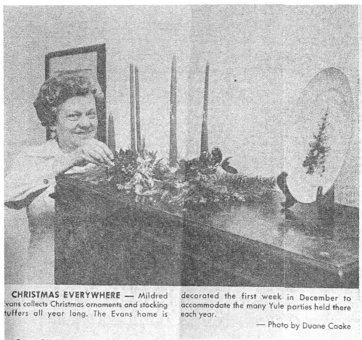

CHRISTMAS EVERYWHERE — Mildred vans collects Christmas ornaments and stocking tuffers all year long. The Evans home is decorated the first week in December to accommodate the many Yule parties held there each year.

— Photo by Duane Cooke

From the Baton Rouge State Times, December 20, 1978

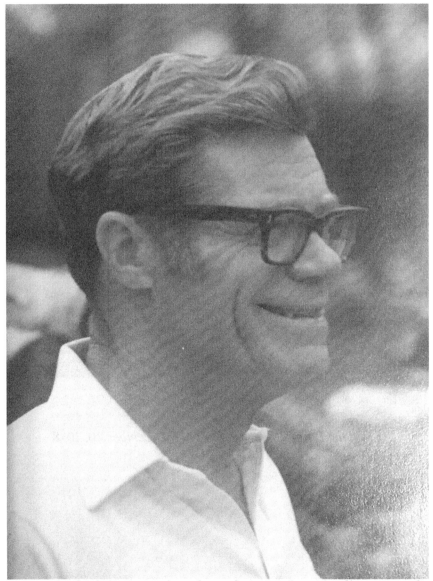

Text on back of picture, written by Red Evans: "W.J. 'Red' Evans, as he appeared any time between Spring 1941 and Spring 1981"

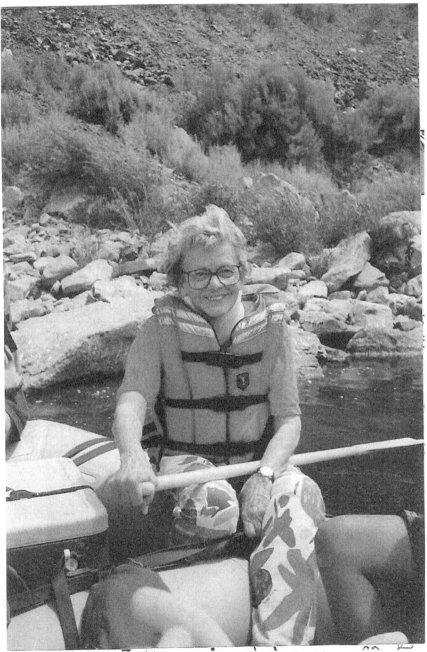

Mildred Evans white water rafting in Colorado c. 1995

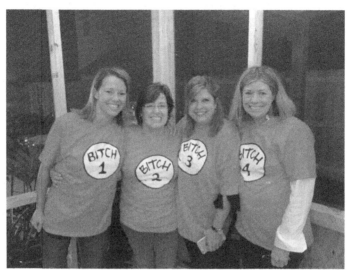

The Four Bees, November 24, 2016

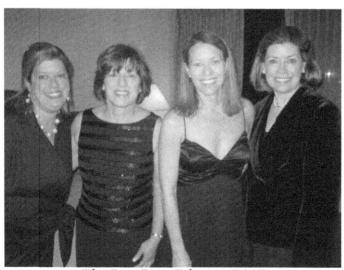

The Four Bees, February 2007

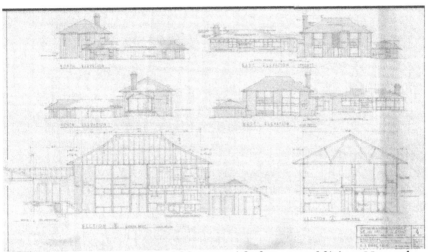

Elevation drawings of the old house with the new addition, November 21, 1969

About the Author

VIRGINIA CAROLINE EVANS IS the sixth child of Mildred and Red Evans. Born and raised in Baton Rouge, Louisiana, she grew up with five older siblings whose ages spanned 22 years. Though her parents were older, they raised her to love LSU football, home-cooked meals, and precious time with her family.

Virginia graduated from LSU in 1991, and LSU Law School in 1996. She has spent most of her career helping clients with real estate, estate planning, and successions; however, she is currently enjoying her position with the Louisiana Department of Justice. She is also looking forward to writing a sequel to *The Youngest Bee* as well as a work of fiction.

When not working, Virginia enjoys traveling to see her family, and attending musicals and plays with her teenaged daughter. She loves sharing her valuable experience as a daughter and caregiver of an Alzheimer's patient and helping others cope with aging parents. She currently lives in Baton Rouge, and has two daughters, a dog, and a cat. She survives by always maintaining a sense of humor.

Made in the USA
Coppell, TX
28 October 2025